# RENAL DIET COOKBOOK & DIET PLAN

2000+ Days of kidney-friendly, delicious and affordable recipes.
A complete and practical guide to meet your taste and dietary needs
+ 90-days Meal Plan

ANGELA HARPER

© Copyright 2025

The contents of this book may not be reproduced, duplicated, or transmitted without the written permission of the author or publisher. Under no circumstances shall the publisher, or the author, be held liable or legally responsible for any damages, compensation, or monetary loss due to the information contained in this book. Either directly or indirectly.

Legal notice: This book is copyrighted. This book is for personal use only. You may not modify, distribute, sell, use, quote, or paraphrase any part or content of this book without the consent of the author or publisher.

# INDEX

| | |
|---|---|
| Chapter 1: Basic Principles of the Renal Diet | 6 |
|     Basic concepts of the renal diet | 6 |
|     Role of Diet in the Management of Renal Disease | 8 |
|     Specific Nutritional Goals for Patients with Renal Disease | 11 |
| Chapter 2: Sodium Management | 14 |
|     Importance of Sodium Control in the Renal Diet | 14 |
|     Tips for Reducing Sodium Intake in Recipes | 16 |
|     List of Sodium-Free Herbs, Spices, and Seasonings to Add Flavor | 18 |
| Chapter 3: Potassium Control | 21 |
|     Limitations on Potassium Intake for Patients with Kidney Disease | 21 |
|     Identification of High-Potassium Foods and Low-Potassium Alternatives | 23 |
|     Culinary Preparation Techniques to Reduce Potassium Content in Foods | 25 |
| Chapter 4: Phosphorus Limitation | 28 |
|     Role of Phosphorus in Kidney Disease and Risks Associated with Excess Phosphorus | 28 |
|     Foods High in Phosphorus to Limit or Avoid | 30 |
|     Tips for Preparing Low Phosphorus Meals | 32 |
| Chapter 5: Moderate Protein Intake | 35 |
|     Importance of Moderate Protein Intake in the Renal Diet | 35 |
|     Recommended Sources of Lean Protein | 37 |
|     Balanced Recipes with Adequate Amounts of Protein | 39 |
| Chapter 6: Balanced Approach to Carbohydrates | 41 |
|     Role of Carbohydrates in the Renal Diet | 41 |
|     Healthy Carbohydrate Choices That Are Low in Sodium, Potassium, and Phosphorus | 43 |
|     Recipes for Balanced and Nutritious Carbohydrate Dishes | 45 |
| RECIPES: Breakfast | 48 |
|     Overnight Oats with Blueberries and Chia Seeds | 48 |
|     Greek Yogurt Parfait with Raspberries and Honey | 49 |
|     Scrambled Egg Whites with Bell Peppers and Spinach | 50 |
|     Smoothie with Blueberries and Low-Potassium Fruits | 51 |
|     Quinoa Breakfast Porridge with Apples | 52 |
|     Whole Wheat Toast with Low-Potassium Vegetables and Herbs | 53 |
|     Egg White Omelet with Mushrooms and Chives | 54 |
|     Cottage Cheese with Low-Potassium Fruit | 55 |
|     Warm Millet Cereal with Almond Milk and Strawberries | 56 |
|     Whole Wheat English Muffin with Almond Butter | 57 |

- Buckwheat Pancakes with Fresh Fruit — 58
- Poached Egg Whites over Arugula and Roasted Red Peppers — 59
- Tofu Scramble with Turmeric and Diced Zucchini — 60
- Berry Smoothie with Spinach and Flaxseed — 61
- Sweet Potato Hash — 62
- Oat Bran Muffins — 63
- Polenta with Low-Potassium Mushrooms and Herbs — 64
- Farina Porridge with Peaches — 65
- Whole Grain Waffles with Coconut Yogurt — 66
- Rice Cakes Topped with Hummus and Herbs — 67
- Lunch — 68
  - Quinoa Salad with Roasted Low-Potassium Vegetables — 68
  - Lentil Soup — 69
  - Grilled Chicken Wrap with Lettuce and Tomato — 70
  - Egg White Salad Sandwich on Whole Grain Bread — 71
  - Salmon Salad with Greens — 72
  - Chickpea Curry — 73
  - Roasted Turkey Sandwich with Cucumber and Mustard — 74
  - Tuna Salad with Bell Peppers — 75
  - Black Bean Salsa with Pita — 76
  - Couscous Salad with Mint and Lemon — 77
  - Chicken Lettuce Wraps with Shredded Carrots — 78
  - Caprese Salad — 79
  - White Bean Stew with Low-Sodium Broth — 80
  - Orzo Pasta Salad with Tomatoes and Olives — 81
  - Zucchini Noodles with Turkey Meatballs — 82
  - Cauliflower Fried Rice with Peas — 83
  - Barley and Beet Salad — 84
  - Sweet Potato and Spinach Quesadilla — 85
  - Rice Noodle Salad with Shrimp — 86
  - Greek-Style Tabbouleh with Parsley and Lemon — 87
- Dinner — 88
  - Baked Cod with Lemon and Dill Over Wild Rice — 88
  - Grilled Salmon with Steamed Low-Potassium Vegetables and Quinoa — 89
  - Herb-Crusted Chicken Breast with Sautéed Zucchini — 90
  - Stuffed Bell Peppers with Ground Turkey and Brown Rice — 91

| | |
|---|---|
| Braised Tofu with Bok Choy and Sesame Oil | 92 |
| Shrimp Stir-Fry with Snow Peas and Jasmine Rice | 93 |
| Chicken and Vegetable Kebabs with Couscous | 94 |
| Mushroom Risotto with Herbs | 95 |
| Turkey Chili with Kidney Beans | 97 |
| Lentil Loaf with Mashed Sweet Potatoes | 98 |
| Grilled Lamb Chops with Roasted Brussels Sprouts | 99 |
| Vegetable Paella with Parsley | 100 |
| Spinach and Ricotta-Stuffed Chicken Breast | 101 |
| Quinoa-Stuffed Acorn Squash | 102 |
| Broiled Flank Steak with Barley | 103 |
| Zucchini Lasagna with Ricotta | 104 |
| Ratatouille with Couscous | 105 |
| Roasted Vegetable Frittata with Baby Spinach | 106 |
| Spaghetti Squash with Turkey Bolognese Sauce | 107 |
| **Snacks** | **109** |
| Apple Slices with Almond Butter | 109 |
| Sliced Bell Peppers with Hummus | 110 |
| Cucumber Rounds with Yogurt-Based Dip | 111 |
| Trail Mix with Unsalted Seeds and Dried Apples | 112 |
| Celery Sticks with Cottage Cheese | 113 |
| Fresh Pineapple Chunks | 114 |
| Whole Wheat Crackers with Guacamole | 115 |
| Carrot Sticks with Tahini | 116 |
| Air-Popped Popcorn with Paprika | 117 |
| Rice Cakes with Sunflower Seed Butter and Pear Slices | 118 |
| **Drink Recipes** | **119** |
| Blueberry Banana Smoothie with Almond Milk | 119 |
| Strawberry Basil Lemonade | 120 |
| Pineapple Mint Iced Tea | 121 |
| Cucumber Lime Refresher | 122 |
| Apple Cinnamon Infused Water | 123 |
| Raspberry Coconut Water Cooler | 124 |
| Ginger Turmeric Tonic | 126 |
| Mango Peach Smoothie with Coconut Water | 127 |
| Herbal Tea Blend with Peppermint and Chamomile | 128 |

# Chapter 1: Basic Principles of the Renal Diet

## Basic concepts of the renal diet

The renal diet is a carefully crafted nutritional approach designed to address the unique and often challenging requirements of individuals with impaired kidney function. Unlike standard dietary recommendations, this plan weaves together strands of science and practicality to help people with kidney disease maintain their health and quality of life. Each component of this diet is thoughtfully considered to align with the specific needs that arise when the kidneys no longer filter blood efficiently, leaving excess waste and fluids in the body. Understanding its principles reveals why this diet is fundamental to managing kidney disease and provides a framework for navigating a path to well-being.

The kidneys are critical players in the body's regulatory system, maintaining electrolyte balance, filtering waste, and excreting excess fluids. However, when they become compromised due to chronic kidney disease (CKD) or acute kidney injury, their ability to fulfill these tasks diminishes. As the disease progresses, toxins can accumulate in the bloodstream, nutrients can become imbalanced, and the delicate interplay of electrolytes like sodium and potassium becomes disrupted. In response to these complex changes, the renal diet emerges as a personalized roadmap, offering a way to lighten the load on the kidneys by minimizing the intake of certain nutrients and emphasizing others that support bodily functions.

The renal diet is anchored by key principles that involve managing the intake of protein, sodium, potassium, phosphorus, and fluids. Protein is a major focus because the kidneys must filter the waste products generated when proteins are broken down. While protein is essential for maintaining muscle mass and supporting bodily functions, an excess can contribute to further kidney damage. The renal diet emphasizes moderate protein intake, often favoring high-quality sources such as lean meats, fish, and eggs, or carefully measured portions of plant-based proteins like legumes and tofu. This approach ensures that the body receives the necessary building blocks while avoiding an overload that could accelerate disease progression.

Sodium management is another pillar of the renal diet. With compromised kidneys, sodium retention becomes problematic, leading to increased fluid retention and hypertension. This exacerbates the strain on the heart and kidneys, raising blood pressure and contributing to complications like edema. To mitigate these effects, the renal diet advises limiting sodium intake by avoiding processed and packaged foods, which are often laden with hidden salts, and by seasoning meals with herbs and spices instead of table salt. This not only supports better fluid balance but also encourages a more mindful approach to eating that involves savoring natural flavors.

Potassium, an essential electrolyte for nerve and muscle function, poses a unique challenge for those with kidney disease. Under normal circumstances, the kidneys regulate potassium levels meticulously. However, as kidney function wanes, potassium can build up in the bloodstream, potentially leading to dangerous conditions like hyperkalemia, which can cause muscle weakness and heart rhythm abnormalities. To navigate this, the renal diet involves avoiding high-potassium foods such as bananas, tomatoes, and potatoes while opting for low-potassium alternatives like apples, cauliflower, and rice. Additionally, specific preparation methods, such as boiling vegetables, can help leach out some of the potassium content, making certain foods safer to consume.

Phosphorus management also plays a crucial role. This mineral, often found in dairy products, nuts, and cola drinks, becomes problematic in kidney disease because it cannot be effectively filtered out. Excess phosphorus can result in bone demineralization and calcification of blood vessels, leading to cardiovascular complications. By limiting the consumption of high-phosphorus foods and being mindful of phosphate additives in processed foods, the renal diet aims to maintain a delicate balance that protects both bones and cardiovascular health.

Fluid control rounds out the foundational principles of the renal diet. With declining kidney function, excess fluid can accumulate, resulting in swelling, high blood pressure, and shortness of breath. In advanced stages of kidney disease, daily fluid intake is carefully monitored to avoid overloading the body's capacity to excrete. Patients are often advised to minimize fluid-rich foods like soups or juicy fruits while savoring their sips to reduce feelings of thirst.

The renal diet also involves a nuanced understanding of individual nutritional needs based on the stage of kidney disease, comorbid conditions like diabetes, and a patient's unique health history. For instance, those on dialysis require more protein due to the loss of amino acids during treatment, while those in earlier stages of CKD may need stricter potassium or phosphorus limits. This intricate balancing act makes collaboration with healthcare professionals essential in crafting a personalized plan that aligns with each patient's needs and lifestyle.

However, the renal diet is not only about restrictions; it's also about fostering a relationship with food that nurtures joy and creativity. Instead of viewing the diet as a stringent rulebook, it can be reimagined as a curated guide that opens up a world of flavors and textures. Herbs like rosemary, thyme, and oregano lend complexity to dishes, while the vibrant colors of peppers, berries, and squash make for visually enticing plates. Recipes can be crafted to embrace global cuisines that naturally align with renal principles, such as Mediterranean-inspired fish with roasted vegetables or a Japanese miso soup with tofu and seaweed.

Furthermore, adopting a renal diet can help patients cultivate new cooking habits that extend beyond kidney health. Avoiding processed foods and choosing fresh, whole ingredients not only reduces sodium and phosphorus intake but also introduces more vitamins and antioxidants into the diet. Preparing meals at home can strengthen family bonds and instill a sense of empowerment and control over one's health journey.

Ultimately, the basic concepts of the renal diet are woven from a blend of science and lifestyle considerations that respect the challenges of living with kidney disease while celebrating the potential for good health through mindful nutrition. It demands careful planning, consistency, and collaboration with dietitians or healthcare professionals. Yet, it promises a future where the delicate interplay between diet and disease is managed gracefully, with each meal offering an opportunity to sustain the body's resilience and elevate the spirit. Through this tailored approach, patients can find solace in knowing they are actively contributing to their wellness while enjoying the simple pleasures of food.

## Role of Diet in the Management of Renal Disease

Diet occupies a pivotal role in the management of renal disease, serving as both a guardrail and a beacon of hope for individuals navigating the tumultuous waters of declining kidney function. When the delicate filtration system within these fist-sized organs falters, the body's once-precise mechanism for regulating nutrients, electrolytes, and waste unravels. Dietary modifications offer a lifeline, a way to stave off the progression of the disease while preserving quality of life. Though this path requires vigilance and adaptation, it illuminates the power of intentional eating in protecting one's health and future.

The kidneys are more than just waste filters. They are essential regulators of the internal environment, maintaining the body's equilibrium by excreting toxins, reabsorbing vital nutrients, and balancing electrolytes and fluids. When renal disease strikes, their function diminishes, leading to the accumulation of metabolic waste and unbalanced electrolytes in the bloodstream. These changes, if unchecked, manifest in symptoms like fatigue, nausea, edema, and hypertension. They also increase the risk of cardiovascular disease, bone disorders, and neurological complications. Here, the importance of a targeted dietary approach becomes evident. By minimizing the intake of nutrients that exacerbate kidney burden and increasing those that protect the body, individuals can slow the progression of renal disease.

Protein intake is a focal point of dietary management. Protein, a macronutrient crucial for muscle maintenance and tissue repair, generates waste products like urea and creatinine when metabolized. In the presence of renal impairment, these byproducts accumulate in the bloodstream, contributing to symptoms such as nausea and decreased appetite. Excess protein consumption further burdens the kidneys, accelerating the disease's progression. However, protein is essential for health, and too little intake can lead to muscle wasting and immune suppression. Thus, striking a balance between sufficient and excessive intake becomes a delicate task. The solution lies in carefully controlling protein portions and choosing high-quality sources like eggs, fish, and lean poultry. This approach ensures adequate nourishment while minimizing the generation of waste.

Electrolyte control is another cornerstone of managing renal disease through diet. Sodium, potassium, and phosphorus must be meticulously managed due to the kidneys' inability to regulate them effectively. Sodium is notorious for causing fluid retention and hypertension, both of which can exacerbate the workload on compromised kidneys and the cardiovascular system. By reducing sodium consumption through the avoidance of processed foods and the strategic use of herbs and spices, patients can better manage their blood pressure and fluid levels. This, in turn, alleviates symptoms like edema and shortness of breath, granting greater comfort and mobility.

Potassium is an essential mineral that supports muscle function and nerve signaling but becomes perilous when levels spike in the bloodstream due to renal impairment. High potassium levels, or hyperkalemia, can result in dangerous heart arrhythmias and muscle weakness. Thus, the renal diet emphasizes avoiding potassium-rich foods like tomatoes, bananas, and potatoes while encouraging low-potassium alternatives. However, managing potassium levels is not solely about avoiding certain foods. The way vegetables are prepared, such as leaching potassium through boiling and discarding the water, can significantly impact their potassium content, allowing for a more varied diet.

Phosphorus, often a silent but persistent threat, can wreak havoc on the bones and cardiovascular system. As renal disease progresses, excess phosphorus can no longer be excreted efficiently, leading to a condition known as hyperphosphatemia. This prompts the body to draw calcium out of bones, causing them to weaken while also contributing to vascular calcification. The result is an elevated risk of fractures and cardiovascular complications. To counter this, the renal diet encourages avoiding high-phosphorus foods like dairy products, nuts, and processed meats, while favoring low-phosphorus options such as certain fruits and vegetables. Furthermore, the increasing prevalence of phosphate additives in processed foods means that patients must become adept at reading labels to steer clear of these hidden dangers.

Fluid management is crucial for individuals whose renal disease has reached advanced stages. With declining kidney function, excess fluids can no longer be efficiently removed, resulting in swelling, increased blood pressure, and respiratory distress. This makes monitoring fluid intake paramount. Patients are often advised to restrict their consumption to a specific daily limit while also avoiding foods high in fluid content, such as soups and ice cream. Flavoring water with lemon slices or drinking small sips frequently can help alleviate thirst without overloading the body. The goal is to maintain fluid balance while reducing the likelihood of complications like pulmonary edema.

Beyond macronutrients and electrolytes, vitamins and minerals play an integral role in managing renal disease. Anemia is a common complication due to reduced erythropoietin production in the kidneys and the frequent dietary restrictions that limit iron-rich foods. Thus, the renal diet must prioritize foods that bolster red blood cell production, such as lean meats and iron-fortified cereals. Similarly, vitamin D supplementation is often necessary, as compromised kidney function inhibits the activation of this vitamin, leading to bone disorders.

Yet, despite these intricacies, the renal diet is not solely about limiting or restricting. It also opens up opportunities for creative and delicious culinary exploration. The artful combination of herbs and spices like rosemary, thyme, and turmeric can elevate the flavor profile of dishes without the need for excessive salt. Low-potassium vegetables such as cauliflower and cucumber can be transformed into flavorful stir-fries and salads, adding a refreshing crunch and color to any meal. Lean proteins like chicken breast or fish fillets can be marinated with zestful combinations of lemon, ginger, and garlic, making each meal a sensory delight while aligning with dietary guidelines.

Dietitians and healthcare professionals become invaluable allies on this journey, guiding patients through the maze of recommendations and helping them tailor their diets to their specific needs and disease stages. For those on dialysis, increased protein intake is necessary to compensate for the loss of amino acids during treatment, whereas early-stage patients may need stricter potassium or phosphorus limits. Personalized diet plans consider each individual's lifestyle, cultural preferences, and health goals, ensuring that adherence feels empowering rather than burdensome.

In this landscape, family and friends can offer support by sharing meals, experimenting with new recipes, and helping patients stay motivated. It's important that those managing renal disease are encouraged to approach their diets with optimism and creativity, as these attitudes can reinforce the therapeutic potential of food. By reframing dietary choices as acts of self-care, individuals can find solace in knowing that each meal is a meaningful step toward managing their health and preserving their future.

Ultimately, the role of diet in managing renal disease transcends mere sustenance. It becomes a form of medicine, fortifying the body against the relentless tide of toxins and imbalances that threaten to overwhelm it. By embracing the principles of the renal diet and collaborating closely with healthcare professionals, individuals can craft a lifestyle that sustains them physically, emotionally, and spiritually. Here, food becomes more than a means to an end; it is a vital tool for restoring balance, promoting resilience, and reclaiming one's agency in the face of illness.

# Specific Nutritional Goals for Patients with Renal Disease

For patients facing the challenges of renal disease, the importance of setting specific nutritional goals cannot be understated. The journey through kidney impairment is fraught with uncertainties and complexities. Still, clear dietary objectives provide a compass, offering patients direction and hope. These goals become the scaffolding upon which individuals can build a sustainable lifestyle that supports both their immediate well-being and their long-term health. By identifying these targets, patients can customize their eating habits to align with the ever-shifting requirements of renal health.

The first nutritional goal is to tailor protein intake to the body's current needs. Protein, an essential macronutrient that builds muscle and repairs tissue, also generates nitrogenous waste products like urea when metabolized. For those with kidney disease, an excess can lead to the accumulation of waste in the bloodstream, resulting in nausea, fatigue, and loss of appetite. However, insufficient protein can also cause muscle wasting and immune system deterioration. For patients not yet on dialysis, the goal is to moderate protein consumption by focusing on high-quality sources like lean meats, eggs, and carefully measured legumes. The precise amount should be determined in consultation with healthcare professionals who consider the patient's stage of renal disease, comorbidities, and overall health. Conversely, those undergoing dialysis require a higher intake to compensate for the loss of amino acids during treatment, ensuring that their muscles remain robust and their bodies resilient.

Equally important is the need to regulate sodium. Sodium, ubiquitous in the modern diet due to its prevalence in processed foods, plays a significant role in exacerbating hypertension and fluid retention. For kidneys unable to maintain fluid and electrolyte balance, this can lead to swelling, high blood pressure, and an overworked heart. The nutritional goal, therefore, becomes limiting sodium intake to levels that prevent these complications while still making meals enjoyable. By favoring fresh, unprocessed foods and using herbs like oregano, thyme, and parsley to enhance flavor, patients can reduce sodium consumption without sacrificing taste. The reward is not only a reduction in blood pressure but also a decrease in the risk of cardiovascular events and improved overall comfort.

Potassium, an essential mineral, is another critical consideration. It is instrumental in nerve and muscle function, but when kidneys falter, potassium levels can rise dangerously, leading to hyperkalemia. This condition can cause severe muscle weakness and disrupt heart rhythms, making it a potentially life-threatening complication. To avoid these risks, patients are encouraged to set specific goals that align with their potassium requirements. This often means limiting high-potassium foods like bananas, tomatoes, and sweet potatoes while focusing on low-potassium options such as apples, cauliflower, and berries. Furthermore, understanding the potassium content of various foods allows patients to enjoy greater variety while adhering to their dietary needs. Cooking techniques like boiling and draining vegetables can also reduce their potassium content, providing a way to safely consume a wider range of foods.

Another crucial objective is managing phosphorus intake. Phosphorus, which is present in many dairy products, nuts, and processed foods, can become hazardous when the kidneys are no longer capable of excreting excess amounts. This leads to hyperphosphatemia, a condition that disrupts bone health and contributes to vascular calcification. The ultimate result is an elevated risk of fractures and cardiovascular issues. By minimizing foods high in phosphorus and learning to recognize the hidden phosphate additives in processed products, patients can better control their intake and protect their bones and arteries. Many healthcare professionals recommend phosphate binders alongside a low-phosphorus diet to ensure optimal management, but it remains critical to be proactive in selecting foods that align with this goal.

The regulation of fluid intake is a paramount goal for those with advanced renal disease. As kidney function declines, fluid begins to accumulate in the body, leading to symptoms like swelling in the extremities, increased blood pressure, and shortness of breath. Setting a specific fluid limit, often determined in collaboration with dietitians and doctors, ensures that patients stay within a safe range that alleviates these symptoms. This may mean minimizing soups, juicy fruits, and other foods high in water content. It also involves strategic sipping throughout the day to keep thirst at bay without surpassing the daily limit. Incorporating lemon slices, cucumber, or herbs into water can add flavor and refreshment while providing patients with a sense of enjoyment and control.

In addition to managing these major nutrients, it's essential to consider the role of micronutrients in supporting overall health. Iron, for instance, is often deficient in patients with renal disease due to dietary restrictions and impaired erythropoietin production. Anemia can sap energy and contribute to cognitive impairment, so the goal should be to consume iron-rich foods such as lean meats, fortified cereals, and leafy greens in combination with vitamin C, which enhances iron absorption. Vitamin D, another nutrient of concern, becomes less active due to compromised kidney function, which impacts bone density and immune health. Supplementation may be necessary to achieve optimal levels and prevent further complications.

Amid these detailed objectives, patients should also aim to cultivate a mindset that embraces creativity and adaptability. Food should not become an adversary but a companion that supports the journey toward wellness. Incorporating a diverse range of herbs, experimenting with global cuisines, and sharing meals with loved ones can transform the process into one of joy rather than obligation. Instead of focusing solely on what cannot be eaten, patients should celebrate the array of vibrant flavors and textures still available to them. The satisfaction of creating a meal that aligns with dietary goals can foster a sense of accomplishment and control over one's health.

Additionally, personalized nutritional goals must consider lifestyle factors, cultural preferences, and psychological well-being. Each patient's needs are unique, and what works for one may not be suitable for another. Tailoring goals to account for a patient's daily activities, stress levels, and social support can ensure that the diet remains realistic and sustainable. When necessary, modifications should be made gradually to allow time for the body and palate to adjust. By remaining flexible and compassionate with themselves, patients can better adhere to their nutritional goals and maintain a positive relationship with food.

Ultimately, the specific nutritional goals of the renal diet serve as pillars of support, offering patients a way to navigate the often-unpredictable landscape of renal disease. They require dedication, knowledge, and collaboration with healthcare professionals, but the reward is a lifestyle that nourishes both body and spirit. With each carefully measured meal, patients move closer to preserving their health, extending their vitality, and reclaiming their agency in a challenging but manageable journey.

# Chapter 2: Sodium Management

## Importance of Sodium Control in the Renal Diet

In the world of renal disease, sodium often emerges as a central villain—a seemingly benign mineral whose excess can wreak havoc on a body struggling to maintain balance. For individuals managing compromised kidney function, sodium becomes more than just a seasoning on the dinner table; it becomes a substance that, if not properly controlled, could unravel the delicate web of health. The importance of sodium control in the renal diet cannot be overstated because, unlike healthy individuals, those with renal disease face an uphill battle when it comes to balancing electrolytes, managing fluid levels, and maintaining optimal blood pressure. Understanding the interplay between sodium and kidney function, and why sodium reduction matters, forms the cornerstone of a renal-friendly lifestyle.

Sodium is a mineral found naturally in various foods and is a primary component of table salt (sodium chloride). In the body, it is responsible for maintaining fluid balance, transmitting nerve impulses, and facilitating muscle contractions. Under normal circumstances, the kidneys carefully regulate sodium levels by excreting any excess through urine. However, when kidney function is impaired, the ability to excrete sodium diminishes, leading to an accumulation that disrupts the body's fluid balance. This disruption often manifests in fluid retention, increased blood pressure, and swelling in the extremities or face. Over time, this cycle of sodium retention and hypertension places additional strain on the kidneys and the cardiovascular system, accelerating the progression of renal disease.

Fluid retention is one of the immediate consequences of excess sodium. The body draws water into the bloodstream to balance out high sodium levels, increasing the overall fluid volume within the circulatory system. This increased volume forces the heart to work harder and raises blood pressure, creating a feedback loop that continues to exacerbate the burden on the kidneys. Edema, or swelling due to fluid accumulation, can also occur in the legs, ankles, and face, leading to discomfort and mobility challenges. In advanced stages, excess fluid can build up in the lungs, causing pulmonary edema, which results in difficulty breathing and requires immediate medical attention.

Hypertension, often a byproduct of fluid retention, remains a significant risk factor for further kidney damage. High blood pressure narrows and weakens the blood vessels in the kidneys over time, reducing their ability to filter blood effectively. This reduction in filtration efficiency allows waste and toxins to accumulate in the bloodstream, increasing the risk of cardiovascular events like heart attacks and strokes. Thus, maintaining sodium control not only prevents immediate complications like fluid overload but also reduces the long-term risks of cardiovascular disease.

Reducing sodium intake becomes paramount to preventing these complications and slowing the progression of renal disease. By lowering the amount of sodium consumed, the body retains less fluid, blood pressure stabilizes, and the cardiovascular system is less burdened. Patients often notice improvements in their energy levels, reduction in edema, and enhanced comfort after reducing sodium, which encourages adherence to this dietary adjustment. It's not just about feeling better in the moment; it's about laying the groundwork for a healthier, more sustainable future.

The importance of sodium control extends beyond the patient's well-being to the practicality of daily life. Processed foods, pre-packaged meals, and restaurant dishes are often laden with hidden sodium. A simple can of soup or a seemingly innocent frozen meal can contain more than half of the recommended daily sodium intake. Learning to identify these hidden sources and make informed choices about what goes into the shopping cart empowers patients to take control of their health. Reading labels becomes a critical skill, as does understanding that phrases like "reduced-sodium" don't necessarily mean "low-sodium." It's a skill that patients and caregivers alike must hone, as even small changes can make a significant impact.

Adapting one's palate is another essential aspect of sodium control. For those accustomed to a high-sodium diet, reducing salt can feel like a deprivation. However, taste buds are remarkably adaptable. Over time, the craving for salt diminishes, and the natural flavors of herbs, spices, and vegetables become more prominent. This shift is not just about avoiding salt but about rediscovering the vibrancy of food. When salt is no longer the star of the show, ingredients like garlic, lemon, and rosemary take center stage, enhancing meals with their aromatic complexity. Creating a new flavor profile rooted in herbs and spices enables patients to enjoy their meals without compromising their health.

Moreover, maintaining a low-sodium diet can inspire creativity in the kitchen. Home cooking allows for precise control over what ends up on the plate, making it possible to experiment with global cuisines that naturally align with low-sodium principles. Mediterranean and Asian flavors, with their emphasis on fresh herbs, citrus, ginger, and low-sodium soy sauces, can transform a simple chicken breast into a culinary journey. Roasting vegetables like peppers, carrots, and zucchini brings out their natural sweetness and provides a colorful backdrop to proteins. By treating food as an art form, patients can explore new culinary techniques that enrich their diet and enhance their lives. Healthcare professionals, particularly dietitians, play an indispensable role in guiding patients through this process. A dietitian can develop a personalized sodium plan that aligns with the patient's stage of renal disease, lifestyle, and taste preferences. They can provide practical tips for cooking, shopping, and eating out that make the transition to a low-sodium diet less daunting. Additionally, regular follow-ups ensure that the patient remains on track and that the plan is adjusted to accommodate changes in health or medication.

However, the importance of sodium control isn't only physiological; it's also psychological. Patients often struggle with the idea of giving up familiar flavors and feel isolated when social gatherings revolve around food. It's vital to reframe this dietary change as an opportunity for growth rather than a restriction. Finding joy in new recipes, sharing meals with loved ones, and celebrating each small health improvement can empower patients to stick with their goals. It's about building a supportive environment where dietary changes are encouraged rather than judged, and where the emphasis is on savoring life rather than simply getting by.

In the grand scheme of renal health, sodium control stands as a critical pillar in a comprehensive approach that integrates nutrition, lifestyle, and medical management. It requires vigilance and a willingness to embrace new habits, but the rewards are immeasurable. Through conscious sodium control, patients can mitigate the burden on their kidneys, protect their cardiovascular health, and preserve their vitality for years to come. In this journey, each carefully seasoned meal becomes a testament to resilience, a statement of intent to live fully despite the challenges of renal disease. By understanding and honoring the importance of sodium control, patients can rewrite the narrative of their health, one flavorful bite at a time.

## Tips for Reducing Sodium Intake in Recipes

Reducing sodium intake in recipes requires a fundamental shift in how we perceive and approach food preparation, especially in a culture where sodium-heavy processed foods and restaurant meals dominate. Sodium, an omnipresent seasoning in many kitchens, is often an unthinking addition, scooped generously or hidden in countless products. Yet, with careful planning and a dash of creativity, it's possible to reduce or eliminate excess salt while still savoring a symphony of flavors in every bite. This practice not only elevates health but also invites an exploration of global cuisines and fresh, vibrant ingredients.

The first and perhaps most crucial tip is to transition away from processed foods and embrace home cooking. Processed foods, including canned soups, frozen dinners, and pre-packaged snacks, often contain hidden sodium additives for flavor and preservation. Cooking from scratch provides control over the ingredients used, allowing for a gradual reduction in sodium levels without sacrificing taste. Start by selecting whole, fresh ingredients and focus on minimally processed foods like vegetables, lean proteins, and grains. This shift makes it easier to modify recipes to your desired sodium levels.

When cooking at home, it's essential to understand that reducing sodium doesn't equate to eliminating flavor. Aromatic herbs, spices, citrus, and vinegars can all contribute to a flavorful, satisfying dish without a single grain of salt. Fresh herbs like parsley, cilantro, basil, and dill offer a burst of freshness when added to salads, sauces, and soups. Spices like paprika, cumin, coriander, and turmeric create complex layers of flavor in roasted meats and stews, transforming an ordinary dish into something exotic. Citrus juices and zest, particularly from lemons and limes, bring brightness to fish, vegetables, and dressings. Vinegars, from balsamic to apple cider, add tang and depth when drizzled over greens or used as marinades.

Layering these flavors is an art, and it starts with marinating proteins or vegetables in herb-based blends before cooking. A marinade of garlic, rosemary, olive oil, and a splash of lemon juice infuses chicken breast with zest and tenderness. Ground cumin, paprika, and coriander can be rubbed onto pork or beef for a smoky, aromatic flavor when grilled or roasted. The acidity of vinegars or citrus juices tenderizes meats and allows the flavors to penetrate more deeply. Meanwhile, adding a hint of honey or maple syrup can counterbalance the acidity and create a more rounded profile.

Another strategy is to incorporate low-sodium or sodium-free broth to create depth in soups, stews, and grains. Commercial broths are often laden with sodium, but homemade broths using vegetable scraps, bones, and aromatic herbs can be simmered for hours to develop a rich, savory base without added salt. To enhance the umami profile, mushrooms, nutritional yeast, and kombu (a type of seaweed) can be added to the broth during cooking. This yields a versatile liquid that can be used in risottos, soups, and sauces.

Gradually adjusting taste buds to lower sodium levels is also crucial. If a recipe traditionally calls for a teaspoon of salt, start by reducing it by a quarter or half, allowing your palate to adapt to the new flavor profile. As the taste buds recalibrate, continue to reduce the amount of salt used in cooking. For dishes that need a final touch, consider finishing with just a pinch of high-quality sea salt or kosher salt at the end to maximize flavor without overloading on sodium.

Textural contrast can enhance the dining experience and distract from the absence of salt. For instance, adding crunchy toasted nuts or seeds to a salad provides a pleasant contrast to leafy greens. Grating fresh vegetables like carrots or radishes into stir-fries offers an unexpected crunch and a subtle sweetness. In pasta dishes, fresh breadcrumbs or a handful of toasted pine nuts can elevate an otherwise simple preparation. Pairing contrasting textures helps create a sense of fullness and satisfaction.

Mindfulness about condiments is also key. Many sauces, ketchups, and dressings are high in sodium, so switching to homemade versions allows for greater control. Homemade ketchup can be made from ripe tomatoes, vinegar, and a touch of honey. Salad dressings can be crafted with olive oil, lemon juice, Dijon mustard, and herbs. Salsa can be whipped up using fresh tomatoes, cilantro, and a dash of lime, avoiding the added salt in jarred versions. Similarly, swapping soy sauce for low-sodium soy sauce or coconut aminos can reduce sodium without compromising on flavor in stir-fries and marinades.

Portion control is an effective way to reduce sodium intake overall. By serving smaller portions of salty dishes and filling the rest of the plate with fresh vegetables or whole grains, it's possible to enjoy a favorite meal without overloading on salt. For example, a small piece of cheese on a salad can add richness and flavor while keeping sodium levels low if balanced with a bed of fresh greens and vinaigrette.

Reading labels becomes essential when purchasing packaged items. Even products marketed as "low-sodium" can have varying definitions, so understanding the specific milligram count of sodium per serving is crucial. Aim for products with no more than 140 milligrams per serving or less than 5 percent of the recommended daily value. Many labels also include "hidden" forms of sodium, such as monosodium glutamate (MSG), sodium nitrate, or baking soda, all of which can contribute to excessive intake. Choosing brands specifically dedicated to low-sodium products can simplify the decision-making process.

Finally, involve family and friends in the journey to reduce sodium. Experimenting with new recipes together, sharing meals, and exploring farmer's markets can foster a shared commitment to healthier eating. With support and encouragement, this lifestyle adjustment becomes less about restriction and more about celebrating the joy of food.

The journey toward lower sodium cooking is a transformative one, requiring patience, experimentation, and a willingness to explore new flavors and techniques. As the palate adjusts to the absence of salt, it becomes easier to appreciate the natural sweetness of roasted carrots, the earthy warmth of cumin, and the crisp acidity of lemon. This shift doesn't just lead to better health outcomes but also enhances the relationship with food, allowing individuals to savor each bite while safeguarding their well-being. Ultimately, reducing sodium intake is a path to rediscovering the authentic, vibrant flavors that nature provides.

## List of Sodium-Free Herbs, Spices, and Seasonings to Add Flavor

Sodium is often thought of as synonymous with flavor, but the truth is that it's only one of countless ingredients that can enrich a dish. Herbs, spices, and seasonings offer an incredible variety of tastes, scents, and colors that elevate any meal while keeping sodium intake in check. Understanding how to wield these ingredients can redefine the concept of flavor and introduce a world of aromatic and healthful culinary possibilities.

Herbs like parsley, cilantro, basil, and mint are excellent starting points. Fresh parsley, with its clean, slightly peppery taste, can be chopped and sprinkled over everything from grilled fish to pasta. Its vibrant green hue enlivens the plate, offering a burst of flavor and color. Cilantro, another fresh herb, adds a distinctive, citrusy note to salsas, marinades, and salads, particularly those with Latin or Asian influences. Basil's sweet, slightly anise-like profile pairs beautifully with tomatoes, cheeses, and olive oil, making it a staple in Mediterranean dishes. Its unmistakable fragrance wafts through the kitchen, promising an unforgettable meal. Mint, which can be chopped into salads, blended into sauces, or infused into drinks, provides a cooling, invigorating taste that contrasts with the warmth of roasted vegetables and grilled meats.

Moving from leafy herbs to woodier varieties like rosemary, thyme, and oregano opens up new avenues for exploration. Rosemary's pine-like aroma and flavor make it ideal for heartier dishes like roasted lamb, chicken, or root vegetables. Its sturdy sprigs can be tied together and used as a basting brush or added whole to a roasting pan. Thyme, with its earthy, lemony undertones, works wonders in soups, stews, and marinades, imparting subtle complexity with each leaf. Oregano, a staple of Italian and Greek cooking, brings a robust, slightly bitter flavor to pasta sauces, pizzas, and dressings. When dried, it can be sprinkled over grilled vegetables, meats, and even eggs to create an herbaceous finish that lingers on the palate.

Spices provide a potent punch of flavor and heat that can transform the simplest ingredients. Ground cumin, with its warm, earthy taste, adds depth to chili, curries, and roasted vegetables. Its aroma evokes faraway markets and ancient culinary traditions, infusing each bite with mystery. Paprika, ranging from sweet to smoked to hot, can be dusted over chicken or fish before grilling or used as a base for spice rubs. Its vivid red hue gives dishes a fiery appearance, even if the heat remains mild. Coriander, the seed of the cilantro plant, offers a subtle citrus flavor that complements fish, rice dishes, and pickled vegetables. Its floral notes are gentle, yet unmistakable, lending an ethereal quality to each dish.

Turmeric, another ancient spice, is known for its brilliant golden color and earthy, slightly bitter taste. Common in Indian cuisine, it can be used in rice dishes, soups, and marinades to bring a vibrant hue and anti-inflammatory properties. Ground ginger, with its pungent, peppery warmth, enhances stir-fries, baked goods, and beverages. Its ability to complement both sweet and savory foods makes it a versatile addition to the spice cabinet.

To elevate the flavors of herbs and spices further, consider incorporating citrus and vinegar. Lemon and lime juices add brightness and acidity to salads, marinades, and roasted vegetables. Their zest—grated or peeled—releases fragrant oils that can be rubbed onto meats or stirred into sauces for an added layer of citrusy complexity. Vinegars like apple cider, balsamic, and red wine introduce tang and sweetness to dressings and glazes, creating a balanced interplay of flavors.

In the quest for umami, nutritional yeast, mushrooms, and seaweed can bring savory richness to plant-based dishes. Nutritional yeast, with its nutty, cheese-like taste, can be sprinkled over popcorn or stirred into soups for a boost of flavor. Mushrooms, particularly shiitake and porcini, are packed with umami compounds that emerge when sautéed or dried and ground into a powder. A handful of dried mushrooms added to broths or sauces imparts an unmistakable depth. Seaweed, especially kombu and wakame, adds a briny, oceanic quality to soups, stir-fries, and even snacks like roasted nori.

Beyond individual herbs and spices, seasoning blends allow for the layering of flavors that enrich any dish. Ras el hanout, a North African spice blend, combines cinnamon, cumin, coriander, and cardamom for a complex, aromatic profile that enhances lamb, chicken, and vegetable stews. Za'atar, a Middle Eastern blend of thyme, sumac, sesame seeds, and oregano, adds a citrusy, nutty touch to pita, hummus, and roasted vegetables. Garam masala, a warm Indian blend of cinnamon, cloves, and cumin, can be stirred into curries or used as a rub for grilled meats.

Incorporating these herbs, spices, and seasonings into your cooking does more than simply replace salt. It cultivates a deeper relationship with the food you prepare and eat, making each meal an opportunity to experiment and indulge in new flavors. By focusing on the scent, appearance, and interplay of different ingredients, a low-sodium diet can transcend the idea of restriction and instead become a celebration of natural tastes.

It is worth noting that adjusting to a salt-free flavor palette requires patience and a willingness to experiment. Start with familiar seasonings and gradually introduce new flavors to allow your palate to adjust. Play with textures and pairings, mixing crunchy nuts with tender herbs or warming spices with bright citrus. Share the results with family and friends, inviting them into your kitchen to embark on this culinary journey with you. As you explore new blends and combinations, you'll find that a diet focused on herbs, spices, and sodium-free seasonings is anything but bland. Instead, it can provide a world of discovery where each bite delights and surprises, proving that salt is just one player in the magnificent orchestra of flavor.

# Chapter 3: Potassium Control

## Limitations on Potassium Intake for Patients with Kidney Disease

For individuals managing kidney disease, controlling potassium levels in the diet becomes a delicate yet crucial balancing act. The mineral potassium, often celebrated for its role in supporting muscle function, nerve signaling, and cardiovascular health, takes on a more precarious position when the kidneys struggle to filter out excess amounts. In healthy individuals, the kidneys maintain a steady level of potassium by excreting any surplus through urine. But with impaired kidney function, this finely-tuned balance falters, and potassium can build up in the bloodstream, potentially leading to a condition known as hyperkalemia, which may trigger muscle weakness, heart arrhythmias, or even sudden cardiac arrest.

The dietary limitation of potassium, therefore, becomes imperative in protecting patients from these life-threatening complications. It requires a thoughtful approach to meal planning and a keen understanding of which foods contain high levels of potassium. Patients, families, and caregivers must work together to identify these foods and make substitutions or adjustments to maintain the enjoyment of meals without compromising health.

Potassium-rich foods, though often nutritious and versatile, must be consumed with caution. Bananas, a popular snack or breakfast staple, are well-known for their high potassium content and are often one of the first foods patients are advised to limit or avoid. Other fruits like oranges, cantaloupe, and avocados similarly pose a risk due to their elevated levels. Vegetables, especially potatoes, tomatoes, and spinach, contain significant potassium, making them problematic in large quantities. Even some grains and legumes, such as bran cereals and lentils, contribute a notable amount of potassium, challenging patients to rethink their typical dietary staples.

However, potassium limitation does not mean abandoning the joy of eating or resigning to a bland diet. Instead, it's about adopting new strategies that safeguard against excess potassium while celebrating a diverse, colorful plate. For instance, apples, berries, grapes, and pineapples are all fruits with relatively low potassium levels, offering sweetness and variety without compromising safety. Vegetables like cauliflower, green beans, cucumbers, and lettuce can provide crunch, color, and nutrition without the potassium overload of potatoes or spinach.

Additionally, the method of preparing food can greatly influence its potassium content. Leaching, a process where vegetables are soaked or boiled and the water discarded, helps to draw out some of the potassium. For instance, potatoes can be peeled, diced, soaked for several hours, and then boiled to significantly reduce their potassium levels. This allows patients to enjoy the occasional mashed or roasted potato without overloading on the mineral. Similarly, vegetables like carrots and winter squash benefit from a brief boiling or blanching to leach out some of their potassium. While this process can alter texture and flavor, it opens up opportunities to enjoy otherwise off-limits foods.

Another critical aspect of managing potassium involves recognizing and avoiding hidden sources. Processed foods, often laden with additives and preservatives, can contain significant amounts of potassium in the form of potassium chloride, potassium citrate, or potassium phosphate. Reading labels carefully becomes essential, as seemingly innocuous items like bread, salad dressings, or canned soups can harbor these additives. Reduced-sodium products may also use potassium chloride as a salt substitute, which can inadvertently increase potassium intake. It's important for patients to scrutinize labels and opt for fresh, homemade alternatives whenever possible.

Dining out presents its own challenges. Restaurant meals often contain high-potassium ingredients or use pre-made sauces and mixes with hidden potassium additives. Patients can navigate these challenges by being proactive—asking questions about ingredients and preparation methods, requesting that sauces or dressings be served on the side, and choosing simple, grilled, or steamed dishes. Many restaurants are willing to accommodate dietary needs if given clear guidance, and patients can build a repertoire of reliable, low-potassium options that satisfy their cravings.

Maintaining potassium control isn't just about restriction; it's also about ensuring adequate nutrient intake. Protein, often necessary in moderate amounts for those with kidney disease, can be found in lean meats, poultry, fish, and egg whites, all of which are low in potassium. Incorporating these proteins into meals alongside low-potassium vegetables and grains ensures that the diet remains balanced. Healthy fats, such as olive oil and certain seeds, can also provide essential nutrients without significantly impacting potassium levels.

The psychological and emotional aspects of dietary changes cannot be overlooked. For patients accustomed to snacking on bananas or digging into a bowl of tomato-based pasta, learning to avoid these favorites can feel overwhelming and isolating. It's vital to approach potassium limitation with flexibility and compassion, allowing room for occasional indulgences and substitutions that keep the diet varied and enjoyable. Experimenting with new recipes and flavors, such as a crisp cucumber and apple salad or a tangy pineapple salsa, can transform the challenge into an opportunity for culinary exploration.

Dietitians and healthcare professionals play an indispensable role in supporting this transition, providing personalized guidance that aligns with the patient's stage of renal disease, lifestyle, and health goals. They can help identify safe portions and substitutions for high-potassium foods and offer strategies for dining out, meal prepping, and adapting favorite recipes. Their expertise ensures that the patient's diet remains safe, nutritionally balanced, and tailored to their unique needs.

Family and friends are also instrumental in fostering a supportive environment. By sharing meals that meet potassium guidelines, exploring farmer's markets together, or trying new recipes, they can make the process feel less like an obligation and more like a shared adventure. For patients, the reassurance that their loved ones understand their dietary needs and are willing to accommodate them can significantly reduce the emotional burden of these changes.

Ultimately, limitations on potassium intake require vigilance and adaptability. Patients with kidney disease must be attuned to their body's needs, the nutritional composition of their food, and the ways they can still indulge in their favorite dishes while safeguarding their health. Though the path is fraught with challenges, it leads to a space where flavor, nutrition, and well-being coexist harmoniously, promising a life where the joy of eating is still very much on the table.

## Identification of High-Potassium Foods and Low-Potassium Alternatives

Navigating the labyrinth of potassium-rich foods can feel overwhelming for patients with kidney disease, given the vast array of seemingly innocuous ingredients that can tip the potassium balance in the wrong direction. With the kidneys unable to filter out excess potassium effectively, dietary vigilance becomes paramount in preventing the dangerous buildup of this mineral. The solution lies not only in identifying foods to limit or avoid but also in finding satisfying alternatives that allow patients to relish a flavorful and varied diet without compromising their health.

Potassium, an essential mineral that supports nerve signaling, muscle function, and electrolyte balance, is abundant in many common fruits, vegetables, grains, and protein sources. However, its benefits can turn perilous when kidney function declines. Understanding which foods are high in potassium and learning to replace them with low-potassium alternatives helps patients curate their meals thoughtfully while maintaining their enjoyment of food.

Bananas, widely known for their potassium content, are often one of the first foods that patients are advised to limit or avoid. While a banana may offer valuable vitamins and fiber, its high potassium levels make it risky for those managing kidney disease. Instead of bananas, patients can opt for fruits like apples, berries, or pineapples, which contain significantly less potassium while still providing natural sweetness. These fruits can be sliced, chopped into salads, or blended into smoothies to offer texture and flavor.

Oranges and other citrus fruits, similarly high in potassium, can be replaced by lower-potassium options like pears, grapes, or canned peaches (drained and rinsed to remove excess syrup). This substitution allows patients to enjoy their breakfast fruit salad or mid-morning snack without worrying about excessive potassium intake. Canned fruits can be particularly useful because they are often lower in potassium than fresh or dried varieties.

Avocados, another beloved fruit packed with healthy fats and nutrients, can present a challenge due to their high potassium levels. Instead of guacamole or avocado toast, patients can substitute cucumber slices or celery sticks dipped in hummus, a creamy, satisfying snack with less potassium. Hummus, made from chickpeas or white beans, also provides protein and fiber, adding to its appeal.

Vegetables, an integral part of any balanced diet, also vary widely in potassium content. Potatoes, tomatoes, and leafy greens like spinach or Swiss chard are often culprits in high-potassium diets. Potatoes, whether baked, mashed, or fried, can be replaced with alternatives like cauliflower, rice, or pasta, which provide a similar starchy base without the potassium overload. Cauliflower, in particular, can be mashed or riced to mimic potatoes, creating a familiar yet kidney-friendly substitute. When roasted or steamed, it pairs well with herbs and spices, making it versatile for any meal.

Tomatoes, a popular ingredient in sauces, salsas, and soups, can be substituted with roasted red peppers, which offer a similar tangy flavor but with significantly less potassium. Blending these roasted peppers with olive oil, garlic, and a splash of vinegar creates a vibrant sauce that complements pasta, fish, or roasted vegetables. Alternatively, patients can explore tomato-free marinara sauces made from carrots and beets, which provide the sweetness and color of tomatoes without the potassium.

For leafy greens like spinach or Swiss chard, patients can instead enjoy lettuce, cabbage, or kale in moderation. These greens can be shredded into salads, added to wraps, or lightly sautéed to create a side dish that pairs well with protein. Napa cabbage and bok choy, often used in Asian cuisine, provide a crunchy texture and mild flavor suitable for stir-fries and soups.

Legumes and grains, though excellent sources of plant-based protein and fiber, can also pose potassium challenges. Lentils, kidney beans, and black beans are particularly high in potassium and should be consumed in limited portions. For those looking to replace beans in chili or salads, cannellini beans or garbanzo beans offer a slightly lower potassium content while still delivering plant-based protein. Rice, quinoa, and pasta are low-potassium alternatives to whole grains like bran cereals, which can be incorporated into casseroles, grain bowls, or side dishes.

Nuts and seeds, popular snacks known for their heart-healthy fats and protein, often carry a high potassium burden. Almonds, pistachios, and sunflower seeds are among the most potassium-rich. Instead, patients can opt for unsalted popcorn, rice cakes, or pumpkin seeds in moderation. Pumpkin seeds, also known as pepitas, can be toasted and lightly seasoned to add crunch to salads, soups, or roasted vegetables.

Dairy products, while providing essential calcium and protein, can be problematic due to their potassium and phosphorus content. Milk, yogurt, and cheese should be consumed sparingly, with emphasis on lower-potassium alternatives like almond or rice milk. Greek yogurt, although high in protein, carries a significant potassium load and may need to be swapped out for coconut yogurt, which is creamy yet lower in potassium.

While replacing high-potassium foods with low-potassium alternatives requires vigilance, it also opens the door to creative exploration in the kitchen. By experimenting with new combinations of herbs, spices, and flavors, patients can develop dishes that are both satisfying and suitable for their health needs. A vibrant cucumber salad drizzled with lemon juice, a cauliflower mash with rosemary, or a pear and berry smoothie can deliver delightful flavors without tipping the potassium scales.

Beyond substitutions, patients can further enhance their potassium control by varying their portion sizes and combining high-potassium foods with lower-potassium counterparts. For instance, half a slice of avocado on a rice cake or a small dollop of tomato salsa on grilled chicken can offer the desired taste while keeping the overall potassium intake in check. Portion control allows patients to savor their favorite flavors in moderation without feeling deprived.

The journey of identifying high-potassium foods and finding suitable replacements is not without its challenges, but it can become a rewarding exploration of flavor and creativity. With guidance from dietitians and healthcare professionals, patients can feel empowered to craft meals that celebrate vibrant, low-potassium ingredients and bring joy back to the table. In this way, potassium control transforms from a daunting task into a pathway toward a healthier, more fulfilling relationship with food.

## Culinary Preparation Techniques to Reduce Potassium Content in Foods

For patients with kidney disease, controlling potassium intake is a cornerstone of dietary management. Yet, the challenge of enjoying flavorful, familiar foods while keeping potassium levels in check often feels daunting. Fortunately, culinary preparation techniques can reduce potassium content in foods, allowing patients to savor their favorite dishes with less risk. By leveraging these methods, patients can strike a balance between dietary safety and the pleasure of a well-prepared meal.

One of the most effective techniques for reducing potassium in high-potassium vegetables like potatoes, carrots, and sweet potatoes is leaching. Leaching is a process that involves soaking and boiling vegetables to draw out excess potassium. To leach potatoes, for instance, they are peeled and diced into small pieces before soaking in a large bowl of warm water for at least two hours, or overnight for optimal results. Changing the soaking water once or twice enhances potassium removal. After soaking, the potatoes are boiled in fresh water for at least 10 minutes before being prepared in the desired way—whether mashed, roasted, or fried. This method can reduce the potassium content by up to 50%, making previously high-potassium vegetables more manageable.

Blanching is another helpful technique, particularly for leafy greens and cruciferous vegetables. In this method, vegetables are briefly boiled or steamed for two to three minutes before being plunged into ice water to halt the cooking process. By boiling the vegetables and discarding the water, some of the potassium content is removed. Blanching can be done with spinach, Swiss chard, broccoli, or cauliflower, allowing these otherwise high-potassium greens to be incorporated into salads, soups, and stir-fries with less concern. The blanching water should always be discarded because it contains the leached potassium.

Another approach to reducing potassium is boiling or double-cooking foods like squash or eggplant. First, the vegetables are peeled, diced, and soaked in warm water for several hours. They are then boiled in fresh water for 10 minutes, drained, and boiled again for another 10 minutes in fresh water to maximize potassium reduction. This double-cooking process helps make high-potassium vegetables safer to eat while still preserving their flavors and textures.

Choosing canned alternatives can also provide a lower-potassium option in certain cases. Canned fruits and vegetables are often lower in potassium than their fresh counterparts because some of the potassium leaches into the canning liquid. However, it's crucial to rinse and drain the canned products thoroughly before consumption to remove excess sodium and potassium from the liquid. This method works well for canned beans, which can serve as protein sources in salads or soups, and for canned fruits like pears and peaches, which can be enjoyed as snacks or desserts.

Fermentation, a traditional method of preserving vegetables, may also reduce potassium levels. While research is still emerging, some studies suggest that fermented foods like sauerkraut or kimchi might have lower potassium content than raw vegetables due to the leaching effect during fermentation. Patients can experiment with making their own fermented vegetables, ensuring they are rinsed well and consumed in moderation.

In addition to preparation techniques, combining high-potassium foods with low-potassium ingredients can dilute the overall potassium content of a dish. For example, a small portion of high-potassium avocado can be mashed and mixed with a larger portion of diced cucumbers and shredded lettuce to create a satisfying yet low-potassium guacamole. Likewise, adding blanched spinach or leached sweet potatoes to a larger base of steamed rice or pasta can reduce the overall potassium concentration while still providing the desired flavors and textures.

Another important strategy is portion control. By reducing the amount of high-potassium ingredients and pairing them with a larger proportion of low-potassium foods, patients can still enjoy their favorites without significantly affecting their potassium intake. For instance, topping a bowl of pasta with a small spoonful of tomato sauce rather than drowning it can still impart the rich, tangy taste without overwhelming the dish with potassium. Similarly, mixing a few slices of banana into a fruit salad filled with apples and grapes provides the desired flavor while keeping the total potassium intake within safe limits.

Mindful seasoning is also key to enhancing flavor without adding potassium. Herbs, spices, citrus juices, and vinegars can amplify the taste of dishes without increasing potassium levels. Basil, cilantro, parsley, and rosemary can be used generously to create aromatic and colorful garnishes, while spices like cumin, paprika, and turmeric add warmth and complexity to soups and stews. Lemon juice or vinegar can brighten salads and salsas, creating a lively contrast that excites the palate.

While reducing potassium content in foods requires a thoughtful approach, it's also an invitation to explore new flavors, preparation methods, and cuisines. Experimenting with unfamiliar ingredients and techniques can reveal delicious new ways to enjoy mealtimes. For example, substituting blanched spinach for raw or adding mashed cauliflower to potato-based dishes can transform them while keeping the flavors familiar and comforting.

Dietitians play a critical role in guiding patients through this culinary journey, helping them identify high-potassium foods and providing practical advice on preparation methods. They can offer tailored recommendations based on the patient's specific health status, cultural preferences, and dietary goals. Collaborating with healthcare professionals ensures that patients are empowered with the knowledge and tools needed to manage their potassium intake without feeling overwhelmed.

Ultimately, the goal is not just to reduce potassium but to cultivate a joyful and sustainable relationship with food. By embracing these preparation techniques and understanding how to balance high and low-potassium ingredients, patients can continue to celebrate the joy of cooking and eating while safeguarding their health. This process is not only about restriction but also about creativity and exploration—discovering that the journey toward a well-managed diet can be filled with flavor, variety, and vitality.

# Chapter 4: Phosphorus Limitation

## Role of Phosphorus in Kidney Disease and Risks Associated with Excess Phosphorus

Phosphorus is a mineral essential for life, playing a key role in maintaining the structure of bones and teeth, synthesizing DNA, and supporting cellular metabolism. It works in tandem with calcium to maintain bone integrity and ensure proper muscle function. In a healthy person, the kidneys efficiently regulate phosphorus levels, excreting excess amounts through the urine to maintain a delicate balance. However, this regulatory process falters in individuals with kidney disease. As kidney function declines, the ability to filter out phosphorus diminishes, leading to an excess of the mineral in the bloodstream—a condition known as hyperphosphatemia.

Excess phosphorus can be highly detrimental for those with impaired kidney function. High levels of phosphorus in the blood stimulate the secretion of parathyroid hormone (PTH), which, in turn, triggers the release of calcium from bones to counteract the imbalance. This response leads to bone demineralization over time, making bones more brittle and increasing the risk of fractures. This process, known as renal osteodystrophy, is one of the most significant complications of chronic kidney disease. In addition, elevated phosphorus can cause calcium to deposit in blood vessels, tissues, and organs, a phenomenon called vascular calcification, which increases the risk of heart disease, stroke, and peripheral artery disease. Calcification can also result in painful skin lesions and interfere with wound healing.

The risks of excess phosphorus extend beyond physical health to psychological well-being. The long-term effects of hyperphosphatemia, such as chronic bone pain, reduced mobility, and cardiovascular complications, can significantly impact a patient's quality of life. Thus, it is crucial to recognize phosphorus's role in kidney disease and take proactive measures to limit its intake, preventing these risks from manifesting.

Phosphorus naturally occurs in many foods, particularly those rich in protein like dairy products, meat, poultry, and fish. Nuts, seeds, legumes, and whole grains are also significant sources. However, an even greater concern is the phosphorus found in food additives, which are used widely in processed foods like soft drinks, frozen meals, and condiments. Unlike naturally occurring phosphorus, which is often bound to other nutrients, phosphorus additives are highly absorbable, meaning they enter the bloodstream quickly and can cause a more immediate spike in blood phosphorus levels.

With these risks in mind, phosphorus limitation becomes imperative for those with kidney disease. Monitoring and managing dietary phosphorus requires an understanding of food sources and how to incorporate lower-phosphorus alternatives without compromising nutrition and flavor. For example, instead of cow's milk, which contains a significant amount of phosphorus, patients can opt for almond or rice milk, which offer calcium fortification with lower phosphorus content. Non-dairy creamers and sherbets can also be suitable substitutes for those who enjoy adding creaminess to their drinks or desserts.

Meat, poultry, and fish should still be included in the diet but in smaller portions. Lean cuts like chicken breast, turkey, and white fish contain less phosphorus than organ meats or shellfish and can be grilled, roasted, or baked with herbs and spices to provide a flavorful protein source. Eggs, while nutritious, have a high phosphorus content in the yolk, so opting for egg whites in omelets and frittatas offers a protein-rich alternative with reduced phosphorus.

In the grain category, whole grains like bran and brown rice contain more phosphorus than their refined counterparts due to the mineral's concentration in the bran layer. Although refining strips grains of fiber and other nutrients, white rice, pasta, and bread can be incorporated into a low-phosphorus diet with balance. Similarly, potatoes and sweet potatoes, which are naturally high in phosphorus, can be replaced with refined grains like couscous or pasta.

When it comes to nuts, seeds, and legumes, moderation is key. Almonds, peanuts, and sunflower seeds, often considered healthy snacks, can be substituted with unsalted popcorn or rice cakes, which contain less phosphorus. In salads and dressings, patients can replace tahini (made from sesame seeds) with a blend of herbs, olive oil, and lemon juice to impart a burst of flavor without adding excess phosphorus. Similarly, chickpeas, kidney beans, and lentils can be substituted with low-phosphorus vegetables like zucchini, cucumber, or green beans in soups and stews.

Processed foods, which often contain hidden phosphorus additives, should be minimized or avoided altogether. Reading labels becomes a vital skill, and familiarizing oneself with terms like "phosphoric acid," "disodium phosphate," and "calcium phosphate" helps identify potential sources of excess phosphorus. Soft drinks, especially colas, are particularly harmful due to their phosphoric acid content and should be replaced with infused water or herbal teas. Sauces, dressings, and condiments should also be scrutinized, and homemade alternatives can offer fresher flavors with controlled phosphorus levels.

Monitoring phosphorus isn't just about reducing intake; it's also about ensuring the body receives enough calcium and vitamin D. These nutrients work in synergy with phosphorus to maintain bone health, and patients with kidney disease often need supplementation. However, vitamin D supplementation should only occur under medical supervision because excessive intake can exacerbate hypercalcemia (high blood calcium), leading to further calcification of blood vessels.

Phosphorus binders, medications that bind to phosphorus in the digestive tract to prevent absorption, can also aid in managing phosphorus levels when diet alone isn't sufficient. They are often taken with meals and should be used in combination with a low-phosphorus diet for optimal results.

Ultimately, the role of phosphorus in kidney disease and the risks of excess phosphorus require a comprehensive approach to dietary management. By recognizing phosphorus-rich foods and understanding how to make suitable substitutions, patients can enjoy meals that are satisfying and nourishing without compromising their health. Collaboration with dietitians and healthcare professionals ensures that these dietary changes are personalized, sustainable, and aligned with each patient's unique needs and lifestyle.

Phosphorus limitation is not about deprivation but rather about protecting bone health, preventing cardiovascular complications, and ultimately fostering a future where individuals with kidney disease can live fully and joyfully. This journey calls for vigilance and creativity, but the rewards—a body strengthened by nutrition and a life unburdened by excess phosphorus—are well worth the effort.

## Foods High in Phosphorus to Limit or Avoid

For patients with kidney disease, understanding which foods are high in phosphorus is crucial to effectively managing the delicate balance required to stay healthy. Phosphorus is a mineral found in various foods that is essential for many bodily functions, such as building strong bones and teeth, maintaining cellular structure, and regulating energy metabolism. However, when kidneys can no longer filter out excess phosphorus due to disease, it accumulates in the bloodstream, leading to dangerous complications like bone demineralization and vascular calcification. To mitigate these risks, patients must identify and limit foods high in phosphorus while discovering alternatives that align with their dietary needs.

Dairy products are perhaps the most well-known sources of phosphorus. While traditionally valued for their calcium content, dairy items like milk, cheese, and yogurt also carry significant phosphorus levels. For example, a single cup of cow's milk contains around 230 milligrams of phosphorus, and certain cheeses, especially processed varieties like American cheese, can deliver even more. Greek yogurt, a favorite due to its high protein content, should also be limited because it contains more phosphorus than regular yogurt. While dairy alternatives such as almond or rice milk offer lower phosphorus levels, patients should choose unsweetened varieties fortified with calcium.

Meat, poultry, and fish, while important sources of protein, also contribute to phosphorus intake. Organ meats like liver and heart contain particularly high levels of phosphorus and should be avoided or consumed sparingly. Shellfish like shrimp, crab, and oysters are similarly high in phosphorus. Instead, opting for lean cuts of chicken, turkey, or white fish in controlled portions can provide protein with a lower phosphorus burden. Cooking methods like grilling or roasting with herbs and spices can enhance flavor while keeping the meal light and nutritious.

Legumes, nuts, and seeds, though often considered healthy snacks or protein alternatives, should also be consumed with care. Chickpeas, lentils, and black beans contain phosphorus levels that could pose a problem if eaten in excess. Almonds, peanuts, and pumpkin seeds, popular for their crunch and heart-healthy fats, are similarly problematic. Instead of nuts and seeds, patients can try unsalted popcorn, which delivers a satisfying crunch without the phosphorus content. When legumes are preferred, they should be cooked and portioned carefully to minimize phosphorus intake.

Grains, particularly whole grains, are another category to approach with caution. The bran layer of whole grains like brown rice, oatmeal, and whole wheat flour contains high concentrations of phosphorus. This makes refined grains like white rice, pasta, and white bread safer choices, as they are lower in phosphorus due to processing. Though refined grains lack fiber and other nutrients present in whole grains, incorporating vegetables, lean proteins, and healthy fats can make meals more balanced.

Processed foods, particularly those with additives and preservatives, represent one of the greatest hidden dangers in terms of phosphorus. Phosphoric acid, a common preservative in cola drinks, enhances flavor while contributing a significant amount of phosphorus. Other additives like disodium phosphate, sodium hexametaphosphate, and calcium phosphate are frequently used in processed meats, baked goods, and condiments. These additives are quickly absorbed by the body, leading to a rapid increase in blood phosphorus levels. Reading labels carefully and avoiding products with these ingredients helps reduce exposure. Instead of store-bought salad dressings or sauces, patients can make their own using fresh herbs, olive oil, and vinegar.

Certain vegetables are also high in phosphorus and should be eaten in moderation. Potatoes and sweet potatoes contain significant phosphorus levels, but their potassium content makes them even more challenging for kidney disease patients. Leafy greens like spinach, Swiss chard, and kale are also high in phosphorus and may need to be limited. Instead, patients can opt for lettuce, cabbage, and zucchini, which offer lower phosphorus levels while still providing vitamins and fiber.

Beverages are often overlooked as sources of phosphorus but can greatly impact intake. Cola drinks, beer, and some energy drinks are particularly problematic due to phosphoric acid content. Dark colas contain significantly more phosphorus than clear sodas, so swapping them for sparkling water infused with lemon or herbal teas can help reduce phosphorus intake while still providing a refreshing drink. Beer, especially dark or stout varieties, should be limited or replaced with low-phosphorus drinks like flavored water or non-alcoholic beer.

While limiting high-phosphorus foods requires vigilance and careful planning, it does not necessitate sacrificing flavor or satisfaction. Learning to identify problematic foods and seeking suitable alternatives allows patients to maintain an exciting, nutrient-rich diet that meets their health goals. For example, pairing white rice with grilled chicken and steamed vegetables offers a hearty, comforting meal without the phosphorus overload of a bran cereal or organ meat. Creating homemade dressings and condiments ensures greater control over additives and reduces the risk of hidden phosphorus.

To further enhance phosphorus control, patients should consider working closely with dietitians and healthcare professionals who can tailor recommendations based on individual needs and preferences. They can provide personalized advice on portion sizes, substitutions, and meal planning to ensure that dietary changes are sustainable and aligned with the patient's lifestyle. With their support, patients can enjoy a diverse array of meals while protecting their bones, cardiovascular system, and overall well-being.

Ultimately, the process of identifying high-phosphorus foods and limiting their consumption is a journey of discovery. It encourages patients to rethink their relationship with food, experiment with new ingredients, and redefine their favorite meals with lower phosphorus alternatives. This journey isn't about restriction or deprivation; it's about empowerment and understanding how to nourish the body in ways that support health and vitality. With a proactive approach, patients can cultivate a vibrant, satisfying diet that not only aligns with phosphorus limitations but also celebrates the joy of eating.

## Tips for Preparing Low Phosphorus Meals

Creating low-phosphorus meals involves finding a delicate balance between adhering to dietary restrictions and nurturing the pleasure of eating. For those managing kidney disease, cooking with phosphorus in mind requires strategic ingredient selection and thoughtful culinary techniques. By integrating these principles into meal preparation, patients can navigate the complexities of their diet while enjoying a diverse, flavorful array of dishes that align with their health needs.

The first step in preparing low-phosphorus meals is to prioritize fresh, whole ingredients. Processed foods often contain phosphorus additives, which are quickly absorbed by the body and significantly raise blood phosphorus levels. Choosing fresh vegetables, lean proteins, and grains reduces the risk of hidden phosphorus while offering greater control over flavors and textures. Vegetables like green beans, zucchini, cauliflower, and bell peppers can be steamed, grilled, or roasted with herbs to create colorful and nutritious side dishes. Lettuce, cabbage, and cucumbers can form the base of salads that can be topped with lean meats or fish, making a light yet satisfying lunch or dinner.

When it comes to protein sources, opt for smaller portions of lean meats, poultry, or fish, which provide ample protein without overloading on phosphorus. Chicken breasts, turkey cutlets, and white fish like cod or tilapia are all versatile choices that can be seasoned with spices, marinated, or rubbed with garlic and herbs before being grilled or baked. For a tangy twist, citrus juices like lemon or lime can infuse meats with flavor while keeping the meal light and refreshing. Cooking techniques like braising or slow-cooking can also tenderize lean proteins and develop complex flavors that make meals more enjoyable.

Eggs, another source of protein, should be used selectively. Egg whites contain minimal phosphorus compared to yolks and can be used to create omelets, frittatas, or scrambles with vegetables like bell peppers, onions, and mushrooms. Adding herbs like chives, parsley, or basil introduces a burst of freshness and color that enlivens the dish. Pairing these egg dishes with a side of steamed or roasted vegetables ensures a balanced meal.

Grains play a pivotal role in the kidney-friendly diet, offering a starchy base that pairs well with proteins and vegetables. While whole grains like brown rice and bran cereals contain more fiber, they also harbor high levels of phosphorus. Opting for refined grains like white rice, pasta, or couscous provides a safer alternative without compromising texture or versatility. For breakfast, white bread or English muffins can be toasted and topped with low-phosphorus spreads like apple butter or a thin layer of fruit preserves.

Avoiding dairy products can pose a challenge because they are not only high in phosphorus but also valued for their calcium content. Fortunately, plant-based milk alternatives like almond, rice, or oat milk offer a lower-phosphorus option while still providing creaminess. These can be used in smoothies, cereals, or even baked goods. Non-dairy creamers can also replace traditional cream in coffee or tea, while sherbet can be a refreshing dessert alternative to ice cream.

Condiments and dressings are another area where phosphorus lurks unexpectedly. Store-bought sauces, salad dressings, and gravies often contain phosphorus additives that quickly add up. Making these condiments at home ensures better control over the ingredients and reduces phosphorus exposure. For a simple salad dressing, blend fresh herbs like basil or cilantro with olive oil, lemon juice, and a dash of vinegar. For marinades, garlic, ginger, soy sauce (low-sodium), and rice wine vinegar can create an umami-rich flavor that works well with meats and vegetables.

Another crucial aspect of preparing low-phosphorus meals is portion control. By serving smaller amounts of high-phosphorus foods and combining them with larger portions of low-phosphorus vegetables and grains, patients can enjoy the flavors they love without exceeding their phosphorus limits. For instance, pairing a small portion of chicken with a larger helping of steamed rice and roasted carrots creates a meal that's both satisfying and kidney-friendly. Similarly, a lean pork chop with a side of pasta and sautéed zucchini can provide a balanced dinner.

In addition to portion control, patients should be aware of cooking methods that can reduce phosphorus levels in certain foods. For example, boiling and then discarding the water helps to leach out some phosphorus from high-phosphorus vegetables like potatoes and sweet potatoes. This allows patients to enjoy these foods occasionally without significantly impacting their phosphorus intake. Blanching leafy greens like spinach can also reduce their phosphorus content, making them safer to include in soups or casseroles.

Meal prepping and batch cooking can also simplify the process of maintaining a low-phosphorus diet. By preparing larger quantities of proteins, grains, and vegetables at once, patients can mix and match ingredients throughout the week to create diverse meals without spending hours in the kitchen. For example, cooking a large batch of grilled chicken breasts or steamed rice allows them to be combined with different sauces, herbs, or vegetables for variety. Keeping chopped vegetables on hand makes it easy to toss them into a stir-fry, salad, or grain bowl.

Ultimately, preparing low-phosphorus meals requires creativity and a willingness to experiment with new flavors and techniques. By embracing the richness of fresh herbs, spices, and whole ingredients, patients can transform simple dishes into culinary delights that celebrate the joy of eating. Collaboration with dietitians and healthcare professionals ensures that these meals are nutritionally balanced, align with individual needs, and provide variety.

While managing phosphorus intake is challenging, it is also an opportunity to reconnect with the kitchen and rediscover the power of home-cooked meals. Cooking with intention and exploring the vibrant world of low-phosphorus ingredients can turn mealtime into a rewarding ritual. Each dish, carefully crafted with health and flavor in mind, becomes a testament to resilience, offering patients the chance to savor every bite while protecting their future.

# Chapter 5: Moderate Protein Intake

## Importance of Moderate Protein Intake in the Renal Diet

Protein plays a vital role in supporting our bodies. It builds and repairs muscles and tissues, helps produce essential enzymes and hormones, and strengthens our immune system. For those with kidney disease, however, protein presents a paradox. It is necessary to sustain life, but when broken down by the body, it creates waste products that impaired kidneys cannot efficiently filter out. These waste products, like urea and creatinine, accumulate in the bloodstream, potentially leading to nausea, fatigue, and loss of appetite. Therefore, understanding the importance of moderate protein intake in the renal diet is crucial for slowing disease progression and maintaining the best possible quality of life.

In healthy individuals, protein metabolism is a seamless process. The kidneys handle the filtration of waste efficiently and consistently. However, in patients with kidney disease, compromised kidney function reduces the organ's capacity to clear these byproducts. The goal of protein management in the renal diet is to strike a balance between consuming enough to maintain muscle mass and bodily functions while preventing the buildup of harmful waste products.

The importance of this balance cannot be overstated. Too little protein intake can result in malnutrition, muscle wasting, and a weakened immune system, leaving the body more vulnerable to infection and reducing its ability to heal. On the other hand, too much protein places an extra burden on the kidneys, accelerating the decline in function and leading to further complications. The precise amount of protein needed varies based on the individual's stage of kidney disease and other health factors, but generally, a dietitian will recommend an intake that aligns with a patient's specific needs and lifestyle.

Patients not on dialysis are often advised to consume less protein than healthy individuals because their kidneys are still responsible for managing protein waste. However, dialysis patients require a higher protein intake to compensate for the amino acids lost during treatment. Regardless of disease stage, the quality and source of protein also play a significant role in how well the body can use it.

High-quality proteins, such as those found in lean meats, eggs, and fish, are complete proteins. They contain all nine essential amino acids that the body cannot produce on its own. Incorporating these proteins into a renal diet provides the body with the necessary building blocks without overburdening the kidneys. Plant-based proteins, such as beans, nuts, and soy products, also offer valuable nutrients but should be consumed in moderation due to their potential potassium and phosphorus content. The key lies in identifying which proteins best meet an individual's unique requirements while maintaining variety and enjoyment in meals.

For patients with kidney disease, moderate protein intake must be combined with other dietary adjustments, such as reducing sodium, potassium, and phosphorus levels. For instance, eggs, a valuable protein source, can be safely incorporated by using only egg whites. This eliminates the phosphorus-heavy yolk while delivering ample protein to support muscle maintenance. Fish, particularly low-phosphorus varieties like cod, tilapia, and haddock, can be grilled, baked, or poached with herbs and spices to provide high-quality protein without an excessive phosphorus load. Lean poultry, such as chicken breast or turkey, can be roasted or grilled and served alongside low-potassium vegetables like zucchini or bell peppers for a satisfying, balanced meal.

Plant-based proteins, while requiring careful portion control, can still be valuable in the renal diet. Tofu, a staple in vegetarian cuisine, offers a versatile protein source that can be marinated, stir-fried, or grilled to create flavorful dishes. Pairing it with low-potassium vegetables and rice provides a light yet filling meal. Quinoa, often considered a grain, is a complete protein with all nine essential amino acids. Although it contains more potassium and phosphorus than refined grains, it can still be included occasionally in small portions to add variety and texture to a meal.

For snacks and lighter meals, Greek yogurt offers another high-protein option but should be chosen carefully due to its phosphorus content. A small serving can be enjoyed with low-potassium fruits like strawberries or blueberries to create a refreshing parfait. Cottage cheese, also high in protein, can be served in moderation with cucumber slices or pineapple chunks for a salty-sweet contrast.

Ultimately, managing protein intake requires not only the right ingredients but also the right mindset. For many patients with kidney disease, transitioning to a moderate-protein diet can feel overwhelming, particularly when familiar meals need adjusting or beloved foods must be consumed sparingly. However, viewing this dietary shift as an opportunity for culinary exploration can transform the process into a journey of flavor and creativity. Experimenting with herbs, spices, and global cuisines opens up new avenues for preparing proteins that excite the palate and satisfy nutritional needs.

It is also essential to build a support network. Working closely with a dietitian or healthcare professional ensures that protein intake is aligned with disease progression and adjusted as necessary. Family and friends can share the journey by exploring new recipes, cooking together, or simply offering encouragement during challenging moments.

Overall, the importance of moderate protein intake in the renal diet cannot be reduced to a simple formula or set of rules. It is a practice rooted in self-awareness, collaboration, and flexibility, requiring patients to understand how their bodies respond to different proteins and adapt their diets accordingly. By prioritizing high-quality proteins, incorporating variety, and seeking professional guidance, individuals can navigate the complexities of kidney disease with resilience and purpose. Every balanced meal becomes a testament to their commitment to health, a reminder that with each mindful bite, they are actively contributing to their wellness journey.

## Recommended Sources of Lean Protein

Choosing lean protein sources is paramount for anyone managing kidney disease through a moderate protein intake. The concept of lean protein emphasizes the quality of protein over quantity, ensuring that each serving is high in essential amino acids while being low in unhealthy fats and unnecessary waste products. Understanding which proteins offer this optimal balance helps patients maintain their health without compromising flavor and variety in their diet.

Lean poultry, particularly chicken and turkey, is an accessible and versatile protein source that can be incorporated into countless dishes. Chicken breast, often regarded as the epitome of lean protein, provides high-quality protein with minimal fat, phosphorus, and potassium. It can be grilled, baked, or poached with herbs and spices to create flavorful meals that suit a wide range of cuisines. For instance, a lemon and rosemary-marinated chicken breast served with roasted carrots or steamed green beans makes a refreshing, low-sodium meal. Turkey breast, similarly lean, can be sliced and paired with cucumber slices or nestled into a whole grain wrap with lettuce for a light lunch.

Fish and seafood provide a bounty of lean protein options with unique flavors and health benefits. White fish like cod, haddock, and tilapia offer high-quality protein with low phosphorus content, making them suitable for kidney disease patients. These fish can be poached in a lemon-garlic broth, grilled with paprika and oregano, or baked with fresh herbs for a satisfying main dish. Fatty fish like salmon, while containing more fat, also provide valuable omega-3 fatty acids that help reduce inflammation and support heart health. A small portion of baked salmon with dill and lemon, accompanied by a mixed salad, offers a balanced meal that's both hearty and refreshing.

Egg whites are another excellent source of lean protein. While egg yolks contain significant phosphorus, the whites provide nearly pure protein without the added mineral load. They can be used to create light omelets or frittatas with a mix of low-potassium vegetables like bell peppers, mushrooms, and spinach. Incorporating herbs like chives or parsley adds brightness and freshness, elevating a simple egg dish into something special. Hard-boiled egg whites can also be sliced into salads or served alongside whole-grain toast for a protein-packed breakfast.

Tofu and tempeh are valuable plant-based proteins that can be tailored to a renal diet when consumed in moderation. Tofu, made from soybeans, is particularly versatile and absorbs the flavors of marinades or seasonings beautifully. It can be stir-fried with ginger and garlic, grilled for a smoky taste, or blended into dips. Tempeh, a fermented soy product, provides a meatier texture and a unique nutty flavor. It can be crumbled into sauces, sliced into stir-fries, or marinated and baked with a mix of low-sodium spices.

Legumes like chickpeas, lentils, and black beans offer plant-based proteins with fiber, vitamins, and minerals. Though they contain higher levels of potassium and phosphorus than other protein sources, they can be safely consumed in small portions. A chickpea salad with cucumbers, lemon juice, and olive oil provides a refreshing snack or side dish, while a cup of lentil soup with herbs and carrots makes a warming meal. Cooking legumes from scratch allows for better control over portion size and seasoning, ensuring that dishes align with the patient's specific needs.

Non-dairy yogurt and milk alternatives provide another source of lean protein that can complement a variety of meals. Greek yogurt made from almond or coconut milk offers a lower-phosphorus alternative to dairy-based yogurt while still delivering a creamy texture and probiotic benefits. It can be topped with berries, sunflower seeds, or a drizzle of honey for a simple dessert. Plant-based milks like almond, rice, or oat milk can be used in smoothies, cereals, or even baking to introduce protein without the dairy-related minerals.

Cottage cheese, though dairy-based, can also be included in the diet in moderation due to its high protein content. A small portion can be enjoyed with a side of sliced pineapple or cucumber, or mixed into salads with diced vegetables for added texture.

Incorporating lean protein sources into the renal diet isn't just about providing essential amino acids but also about cultivating a positive and creative relationship with food. It involves exploring different marinades, experimenting with fresh herbs, and combining complementary ingredients that highlight the unique flavors of each protein. For example, a miso-marinated cod served with steamed bok choy and rice becomes a journey through Asian flavors, while grilled turkey breast with lemon and thyme evokes the Mediterranean.

Building a supportive community also encourages exploring new sources of lean protein. Family and friends can share recipes, cook together, and sample different cuisines that align with dietary goals. Dietitians can provide personalized guidance on portion sizes and offer creative suggestions for pairing proteins with other kidney-friendly ingredients. This network ensures that patients feel empowered in their journey and that each meal becomes an opportunity to celebrate their health and resilience.

Ultimately, the recommended sources of lean protein provide patients with a foundation upon which they can build a vibrant, satisfying diet that not only sustains their health but also celebrates the joy of cooking and eating. Whether it's a simple poached chicken breast with steamed broccoli or a herb-crusted salmon fillet with quinoa, every carefully prepared meal becomes a reminder that a renal diet need not be a restriction but a pathway to culinary discovery. With each new recipe, patients expand their palates, refine their skills, and nurture their well-being, savoring the knowledge that the food they consume contributes directly to their vitality and quality of life.

## Balanced Recipes with Adequate Amounts of Protein

Balancing protein intake in the renal diet requires careful consideration to meet nutritional needs without overburdening the kidneys. Crafting balanced recipes with adequate protein helps patients manage their health while enjoying varied and satisfying meals. The key lies in pairing lean proteins with complementary grains, vegetables, and flavors that create a complete and nourishing plate.

A grilled lemon-garlic chicken breast, for instance, offers an elegant and versatile base for various meals. To make it, marinate boneless chicken breasts in a mix of lemon juice, garlic, olive oil, and thyme, letting the citrus and herbs permeate the meat. Grill the chicken on medium heat until tender and juicy, serving it with a side of steamed asparagus or sautéed zucchini and a portion of brown rice or couscous. The lean chicken provides a high-quality protein source, while the fresh herbs and lemon add brightness. The vegetables and grain deliver fiber and essential nutrients, creating a balanced meal that feels both hearty and light.

For a seafood alternative, consider a baked cod with herbed quinoa. Cod, a mild white fish, pairs beautifully with a blend of herbs like parsley, dill, and basil. Season the fish with these herbs, a sprinkle of paprika, and lemon zest before baking it in a parchment-lined dish with a splash of olive oil. While the cod bakes, prepare a side of quinoa seasoned with lemon juice and finely chopped herbs. Steam a medley of low-potassium vegetables like green beans and carrots to accompany the dish, creating a colorful and balanced meal that aligns with renal diet needs. The flaky cod offers lean protein, while quinoa provides a plant-based protein with all nine essential amino acids.

Vegetarian options can also meet protein requirements with careful planning. A tofu stir-fry with ginger and garlic is a versatile way to incorporate plant-based protein. Press firm tofu to remove excess moisture, then cut it into cubes and marinate it in a mix of soy sauce, ginger, and sesame oil. Sear the tofu cubes in a hot pan until golden brown, then remove them and stir-fry a mix of sliced bell peppers, onions, and bok choy in the same pan. Add the tofu back into the pan, tossing everything with a dash of low-sodium soy sauce or tamari. Serve the stir-fry over a bed of steamed rice, garnished with fresh cilantro and sesame seeds for added flavor. This dish combines the umami richness of tofu with the crispness of vegetables and the warmth of ginger.

Another vegetarian option that can be tailored to a renal diet is a chickpea and cucumber salad. Drain and rinse a can of chickpeas to reduce sodium, then toss them with diced cucumber, cherry tomatoes, and parsley. Dress the salad with a simple mix of lemon juice, olive oil, and a pinch of cumin for earthiness. The chickpeas provide protein and fiber, while the cucumber adds a refreshing crunch. This salad can be enjoyed on its own or served as a side dish with grilled fish or chicken for a more substantial meal.

Eggs, when carefully portioned, can also create protein-rich meals. An egg white omelet filled with low-potassium vegetables is a flavorful and kidney-friendly option. Whisk together egg whites with a splash of water or milk and pour them into a non-stick skillet. Add fillings like diced bell peppers, mushrooms, and spinach, then fold the omelet in half once the eggs have set. Serve the omelet with a side of whole wheat toast and a dollop of cottage cheese for extra protein. Fresh herbs like chives or parsley add brightness, and a slice of tomato or avocado provides balance.

Greek yogurt, though higher in phosphorus than other dairy products, can still be included in moderation. A parfait made from Greek yogurt and berries delivers protein, probiotics, and antioxidants. Layer the yogurt with strawberries, blueberries, and a sprinkle of sunflower seeds or almonds for crunch. This makes for a delightful breakfast or snack that pairs well with a cup of herbal tea or a glass of almond milk.

For a hearty dinner option, consider turkey meatballs with spaghetti squash. Mix ground turkey with finely chopped onion, garlic, parsley, and a pinch of oregano, then shape the mixture into meatballs. Bake them on a lined sheet until golden brown. Meanwhile, halve a spaghetti squash and roast it in the oven until the flesh becomes tender and can be scraped into spaghetti-like strands. Serve the turkey meatballs over the spaghetti squash, topped with a simple marinara sauce made from fresh tomatoes, basil, and garlic. This dish brings together lean protein from the turkey, fiber from the squash, and bright flavors from the herbs and tomatoes.

By crafting balanced recipes that feature high-quality proteins and complementing them with grains, vegetables, and spices, patients can enjoy meals that are as nourishing as they are delicious. This approach not only meets dietary requirements but also transforms the kitchen into a space of creativity and joy, where ingredients become building blocks for vibrant, flavorful meals. Through this process, patients can savor every bite while knowing that their food choices align with their health goals.

# Chapter 6: Balanced Approach to Carbohydrates

## Role of Carbohydrates in the Renal Diet

Carbohydrates have a multifaceted role in the renal diet, offering not only the primary energy source for the body but also a way to bring comfort and joy to the dining table. For patients with kidney disease, navigating the complex world of carbohydrates requires a nuanced approach that balances the need for energy with the necessity of controlling sodium, potassium, and phosphorus intake. By understanding the role of carbohydrates and incorporating them thoughtfully into meals, individuals can support their health while enjoying the variety and flavor these foods bring.

In healthy individuals, carbohydrates serve as the body's preferred energy source. They are broken down into glucose, which fuels the brain, muscles, and other tissues. For patients with chronic kidney disease (CKD), carbohydrates are no less important, but their selection requires a more strategic approach. This is especially relevant for those with diabetes and CKD, as blood sugar control becomes crucial in managing both conditions.

One primary role of carbohydrates in the renal diet is to act as a substitute for proteins and fats, which can be taxing on compromised kidneys. By providing energy through a controlled intake of carbohydrates, patients can reduce their reliance on proteins, minimizing the buildup of waste products like urea that overburden the kidneys. This substitution helps maintain muscle mass and provides fuel for daily activities without exacerbating the decline in kidney function. Carbohydrates also play a significant role in meal satisfaction, offering familiar flavors and textures that provide comfort and promote adherence to the dietary plan.

Choosing the right types of carbohydrates is crucial. Not all carbohydrates are created equal, and their quality and nutritional composition can vary significantly. Simple carbohydrates, like those found in refined sugars and white flour, can lead to rapid blood sugar spikes and provide little nutritional value. Complex carbohydrates, however, offer more sustained energy due to their fiber content and slower digestion rates. They also often come packed with vitamins, minerals, and antioxidants that support overall health.

However, patients must also navigate the potassium and phosphorus content found in many carbohydrate-rich foods. For instance, whole grains, while rich in fiber and nutrients, can harbor higher levels of phosphorus and potassium. To strike the right balance, patients should focus on refined grains like white rice, pasta, and couscous, which contain lower amounts of these minerals while still providing energy. These grains can be fortified with vitamins and minerals to ensure that patients receive adequate nutrition.

Beyond grains, other carbohydrate-rich foods like fruits and vegetables require careful consideration due to their varying potassium content. Apples, berries, grapes, and pineapples are low-potassium fruits that can be enjoyed fresh or cooked into sauces and desserts. Similarly, low-potassium vegetables like green beans, cucumbers, and cabbage can be incorporated into salads, stir-fries, and soups to provide fiber, vitamins, and minerals without significantly impacting potassium intake. These fruits and vegetables complement carbohydrate-rich grains, creating balanced dishes that are colorful, flavorful, and nutrient-dense.

Legumes, such as chickpeas and lentils, offer plant-based carbohydrates with fiber and protein. However, they also contain significant potassium and phosphorus, so patients should consume them in moderation. Instead of making legumes the primary ingredient, they can be used sparingly as toppings or mixed with low-potassium vegetables and grains to dilute their impact. For example, a couscous salad with a small handful of chickpeas and a mix of chopped cucumbers, tomatoes, and parsley provides a vibrant side dish that aligns with renal diet requirements.

Another role carbohydrates play in the renal diet is promoting gut health. Fiber, particularly from complex carbohydrates like grains, fruits, and vegetables, supports digestion and regularity. This is crucial for patients with CKD, as constipation can exacerbate symptoms and make the diet harder to follow. Fiber also helps regulate blood sugar levels, reducing the risk of sudden spikes that can strain the kidneys further. By including a variety of fiber-rich carbohydrates in their diet, patients can support digestive health while enjoying a more satisfying meal.

Carbohydrates also provide versatility and adaptability in the kitchen. Rice, pasta, and bread can serve as the base for countless dishes, each with its own flavor profile. For instance, white rice can be steamed and paired with grilled chicken and roasted vegetables for a light yet hearty meal. Pasta can be tossed with a tomato and basil sauce, accompanied by a side of steamed green beans, for an Italian-inspired dinner. Bread can be toasted and topped with apple butter or a slice of pear for breakfast. These simple yet comforting dishes make it easier to adhere to the renal diet while ensuring that patients receive balanced nutrition.

Sweet potatoes and regular potatoes can also fit into the renal diet when prepared thoughtfully. By peeling, soaking, and boiling them before consumption, patients can significantly reduce their potassium content. Mashed potatoes or roasted sweet potato wedges can then be paired with lean proteins like chicken or fish for a comforting meal that aligns with dietary guidelines.

Overall, the role of carbohydrates in the renal diet extends beyond providing energy. They form the foundation of satisfying meals that support kidney health while offering comfort and pleasure. By selecting high-quality carbohydrates that align with nutritional requirements and complementing them with lean proteins and colorful vegetables, patients can craft meals that not only nurture their bodies but also uplift their spirits. Cooking with intention and exploring new ways to prepare carbohydrate-rich foods encourages creativity in the kitchen and allows patients to redefine their relationship with food, turning every meal into an opportunity for nourishment and joy.

## Healthy Carbohydrate Choices That Are Low in Sodium, Potassium, and Phosphorus

In the world of nutrition, carbohydrates often emerge as comforting staples that bring a sense of familiarity and satisfaction to our daily meals. For patients with kidney disease, however, making carbohydrate choices requires an extra layer of consideration, particularly around the intake of sodium, potassium, and phosphorus. Fortunately, a variety of carbohydrate-rich foods offer nourishing flavors without overloading the body with these minerals. Identifying and incorporating these low-sodium, low-potassium, and low-phosphorus carbohydrates ensures a balanced approach to meals while providing a sense of joy at the table.

One of the first carbohydrate choices worth considering is white rice, a grain that fits seamlessly into many cultural cuisines and dietary preferences. Unlike brown rice or other whole grains, white rice has lower levels of potassium and phosphorus due to the removal of the bran layer during processing. This makes it a safer carbohydrate option for patients with kidney disease. Whether steamed and served alongside lean proteins or sautéed with vegetables for a quick stir-fry, white rice offers a versatile base that can be tailored to any palate. Jasmine or basmati rice can also bring subtle aromatic nuances to dishes, while sushi rice provides a sticky, satisfying texture that works well in wraps or rice bowls.

Pasta, particularly made from refined flour, is another low-potassium carbohydrate that pairs well with various sauces, herbs, and proteins. A plate of spaghetti or penne topped with a light tomato-basil sauce can be a delightful meal without excessive sodium or potassium. Pairing pasta with steamed or roasted vegetables like cauliflower, zucchini, or green beans creates a colorful and balanced dish that aligns with renal diet guidelines. For added variety, pasta salads can be made with a blend of low-potassium vegetables and a light vinaigrette, offering a refreshing and easy-to-pack lunch option.

Couscous, a type of semolina wheat granule, provides a quick-cooking alternative to pasta and rice. Its mild flavor and fluffy texture allow it to absorb the essence of broths, dressings, and marinades, making it an excellent base for salads or warm pilafs. Couscous can be prepared with vegetable broth and mixed with diced cucumber, tomatoes, and parsley for a Mediterranean-inspired side dish. Alternatively, it can be served warm alongside grilled chicken or fish, seasoned with spices like cumin, coriander, and paprika for a North African twist.

Bread, when chosen carefully, can also be part of a renal-friendly diet. White bread, English muffins, and tortillas are often lower in potassium and phosphorus than whole wheat options. Toasted slices of white bread or English muffins can be topped with fruit preserves, apple butter, or a thin layer of low-sodium nut butter for a quick breakfast or snack. Tortillas can wrap up a mix of grilled vegetables and lean meats to create portable, kidney-friendly wraps. For those who enjoy baking, making bread at home provides greater control over sodium content while adding a comforting aroma to the kitchen.

For those seeking gluten-free options, rice noodles offer a low-potassium alternative to wheat-based pasta. These translucent noodles cook quickly and can be tossed into soups, stir-fries, or salads. Pairing them with low-sodium soy sauce, ginger, and sesame oil creates a light and fragrant base that complements proteins like chicken or shrimp. A cold noodle salad with shredded cucumber, carrots, and a splash of rice vinegar provides a refreshing meal for warm days.

Fruits and vegetables, naturally low in sodium, provide another essential source of carbohydrates. Apples, grapes, berries, and pineapples are all low-potassium fruits that can be enjoyed fresh or cooked into sauces, compotes, or desserts. A warm apple compote with a hint of cinnamon can be spooned over toast or stirred into oatmeal, while a simple fruit salad made from berries and grapes adds a burst of sweetness to any meal.

Among vegetables, cauliflower, green beans, cabbage, and lettuce stand out for their low potassium and phosphorus content. Cauliflower can be roasted, mashed, or riced to create a versatile base for stir-fries or casseroles. Green beans and cabbage can be steamed or sautéed with garlic and olive oil for a quick side dish, while lettuce can be shredded into salads or used as a wrap for proteins.

Legumes, though generally high in potassium and phosphorus, can still be included in small portions as long as they are balanced with other low-potassium ingredients. A chickpea and cucumber salad, or a lentil soup with onions and herbs, can provide a plant-based protein option that complements grains and vegetables. By diluting the legumes with low-potassium vegetables and grains, patients can still enjoy these comforting ingredients without exceeding their mineral limits.

Root vegetables like sweet potatoes and regular potatoes can also be included with careful preparation. Peeling, soaking, and boiling these vegetables significantly reduces their potassium levels. This makes them suitable for occasional mashed potatoes, baked sweet potato wedges, or potato salads that bring a sense of warmth and homestyle comfort.

Overall, these carbohydrate choices offer a world of flavors and textures that invite exploration and creativity. By mixing and matching them with lean proteins and fresh herbs, patients can create meals that meet their dietary needs while being flavorful and visually appealing. For example, a bowl of jasmine rice with grilled chicken and steamed green beans can evoke the flavors of Southeast Asia, while a plate of couscous with roasted vegetables and cumin offers a North African flair.

Exploring new ways to prepare these carbohydrates also encourages mindfulness in the kitchen. Roasting vegetables with spices, tossing grains with vinaigrette, or pairing pasta with herbs creates layers of flavor that transform simple ingredients into satisfying dishes. This approach not only ensures that meals remain exciting and enjoyable but also strengthens the patient's connection to the act of cooking and the joy it brings.

Ultimately, incorporating healthy carbohydrate choices that are low in sodium, potassium, and phosphorus requires intention and curiosity. By discovering the possibilities within these ingredients, patients can craft meals that align with their dietary goals while celebrating the vibrant tastes of grains, fruits, and vegetables. Every bowl of rice, plate of pasta, or fruit salad becomes an affirmation of health and vitality, a reminder that food can nurture the body and uplift the spirit even in the face of dietary limitations.

### Recipes for Balanced and Nutritious Carbohydrate Dishes

Crafting balanced and nutritious carbohydrate dishes within the confines of a renal diet requires creativity and care. When thoughtfully paired with lean proteins, herbs, and fresh vegetables, these carbohydrate-based meals can offer a delightful and satisfying experience while adhering to dietary restrictions. Each recipe should honor the principle of moderation and variety, allowing patients to savor flavors from around the globe while managing their sodium, potassium, and phosphorus intake.

A Mediterranean-inspired couscous salad embodies the region's light, aromatic cuisine. To make this refreshing dish, prepare the couscous by combining one cup of the granules with equal parts boiling vegetable broth. Allow it to sit for five minutes, then fluff with a fork. While the couscous rests, dice cucumber, cherry tomatoes, and red onion into small, even pieces. Toss the vegetables with chopped parsley and mint in a bowl, adding a drizzle of olive oil and lemon juice for acidity. Mix in the couscous and finish with a pinch of cumin and coriander for warmth. This salad can be served as a standalone lunch or a side dish with grilled chicken or fish. The couscous provides a light base that absorbs the herbaceous vinaigrette, while the cucumber and mint lend a crisp contrast.

For those seeking something heartier, a baked potato casserole offers a comforting yet kidney-friendly dish. Begin by peeling and slicing russet potatoes into thin rounds, then soak them in water for at least two hours to reduce potassium levels. After draining, layer the potatoes in a greased baking dish. Create a white sauce by melting unsalted butter in a pan, then whisk in a spoonful of flour to form a roux. Gradually stir in rice milk or almond milk, allowing the mixture to thicken. Season the sauce with a dash of nutmeg and thyme before pouring it over the potato layers. Bake the casserole at 375°F until the potatoes are tender and the sauce bubbles, about 45 minutes. This creamy dish can be enjoyed with steamed green beans or a side of coleslaw, providing both warmth and satisfaction without excessive sodium or potassium.

Pasta, a staple of Italian cuisine, can be transformed into a kidney-friendly meal with the right ingredients. A simple spaghetti with lemon-basil sauce is both vibrant and refreshing. Boil the pasta in a large pot of unsalted water, then drain and set aside. In a skillet, heat a few tablespoons of olive oil and add minced garlic and lemon zest. Sauté gently until the garlic is fragrant, then stir in a handful of torn basil leaves. Toss the pasta in the skillet to coat, squeezing fresh lemon juice over the noodles for brightness. Serve the pasta with a side of sautéed zucchini or a mixed salad of romaine and cucumber, balancing the meal with a burst of fresh flavors. The basil and lemon infuse the pasta with a summery aroma, while the sautéed zucchini provides a tender complement.

For breakfast, overnight oats deliver a nutrient-packed and easily customizable option. In a jar, combine rolled oats with almond or coconut milk, a spoonful of chia seeds, and a dash of cinnamon. Stir in diced apples or blueberries for natural sweetness. Seal the jar and refrigerate overnight, allowing the oats to absorb the milk and swell into a creamy pudding-like texture. The next morning, top the oats with a drizzle of honey or a dollop of Greek yogurt for extra protein. This breakfast is perfect for those on the go, providing energy and fiber without requiring cooking time in the morning.

A comforting rice and vegetable stir-fry brings together simple ingredients in a flavorful harmony. Cook white rice according to package instructions and set aside. In a wok or large skillet, heat sesame oil over medium-high heat and add minced garlic and ginger. Stir in diced carrots, snap peas, and sliced mushrooms, tossing until the vegetables are tender-crisp. Add the rice to the pan, drizzling low-sodium soy sauce or tamari over the mixture and tossing to combine. Garnish with scallions and sesame seeds, serving the stir-fry with a side of steamed broccoli. The rice absorbs the nutty sesame oil and soy sauce, while the vegetables retain their texture and color.

A sweet and tangy pineapple quinoa salad offers a tropical twist on traditional grain dishes. Rinse quinoa thoroughly, then cook it in a pot of unsalted water until the grains are fluffy and tender. Once cooled, transfer the quinoa to a bowl and stir in pineapple chunks, diced bell pepper, and chopped cilantro. Dress the salad with a mixture of lime juice, olive oil, and a hint of honey. The result is a refreshing dish that pairs well with grilled shrimp or chicken skewers, making it ideal for summer picnics or light lunches.

For those with a sweet tooth, a baked pear dessert provides natural sweetness without relying on refined sugar. Slice ripe pears in half and remove the cores, then place them in a baking dish. Drizzle the pears with honey and sprinkle them with cinnamon and nutmeg. Add a splash of apple juice to the dish and bake at 350°F until the pears are tender and caramelized. Serve them warm with a dollop of Greek yogurt or a spoonful of almond butter for a balanced dessert that satisfies cravings without excessive sugar or phosphorus.

These recipes demonstrate the limitless possibilities of balanced and nutritious carbohydrate dishes. By pairing grains with fresh vegetables and incorporating natural herbs, spices, and lean proteins, each dish becomes a celebration of flavor and creativity. The flexibility of these ingredients invites experimentation and exploration, empowering patients to transform their meals into moments of nourishment and joy. With intention and curiosity, they can craft dishes that both meet their dietary needs and reflect their unique tastes, proving that a renal diet can be as delightful and diverse as any other.

# RECIPES: Breakfast

## Overnight Oats with Blueberries and Chia Seeds

- **Preparation Time:** 5 minutes (plus overnight chilling)
- **Servings:** 2

**Ingredients:**

- 1 cup (240 ml) unsweetened almond milk
- ½ cup (50 g) rolled oats
- 2 tbsp (30 ml) chia seeds
- ¼ tsp (1.25 ml) vanilla extract
- ½ tsp (2.5 ml) cinnamon
- ½ cup (75 g) fresh blueberries
- 1 tbsp (15 ml) honey (optional)

**Nutritional Values (per serving):**

Calories: 180 Protein: 5 g Carbohydrates: 35 g Fat: 5 g Sodium: 75 mg Potassium: 150 mg Phosphorus: 80 mg

**Procedure:**

1. **Combine Ingredients:** In a medium-sized jar or bowl, combine the almond milk, rolled oats, chia seeds, vanilla extract, and cinnamon. Stir well to ensure even distribution.
2. **Mix & Sweeten:** Add the honey if desired, stirring again to blend the ingredients thoroughly.
3. **Cover & Chill:** Seal the jar or cover the bowl with a lid or plastic wrap. Place it in the refrigerator to chill overnight or for at least 4 hours, allowing the oats and chia seeds to absorb the liquid and soften.
4. **Finish & Serve:** In the morning, give the mixture a quick stir, add the fresh blueberries on top, and enjoy!

**Batch Cooking and Meal Prepping Tips:**

- **Multiple Servings:** Prepare multiple jars or containers of overnight oats at once, so you have breakfast ready for the entire week. This method ensures a nutritious meal is easily accessible.
- **Ingredient Variations:** Substitute or add other kidney-friendly fruits like strawberries or raspberries to vary the flavors.
- **Storage:** Overnight oats can be stored in the refrigerator for up to five days, which makes them an ideal meal-prepping choice for busy individuals.

# Greek Yogurt Parfait with Raspberries and Honey

- **Preparation Time:** 5 minutes
- **Servings:** 2

Ingredients:

- 1½ cups (350 g) Greek yogurt (preferably low-fat or non-fat)
- 1 cup (125 g) fresh raspberries
- 2 tbsp (30 ml) honey
- ¼ cup (25 g) granola or muesli, low-sodium
- 2 tbsp (30 ml) chia seeds (optional for added fiber)

**Nutritional Values (per serving):**

Calories: 220 Protein: 10 g Carbohydrates: 35 g Fat: 5 g Sodium: 65 mg Potassium: 200 mg Phosphorus: 100 mg

**Procedure:**

1. **Prepare Ingredients:** Rinse the raspberries thoroughly and set them aside.
2. **Layer Parfait:** In two glasses or bowls, evenly layer the Greek yogurt, adding half of the portion to each container.
3. **Add Granola and Seeds:** Sprinkle a layer of granola or muesli, followed by a sprinkle of chia seeds, if desired.
4. **Top with Raspberries:** Divide the raspberries evenly between the two servings, placing them on top of the granola and chia seeds.
5. **Drizzle Honey:** Finish the parfaits with a generous drizzle of honey over the top.
6. **Serve Immediately:** The parfaits are best served right after assembly to maintain the granola's crispness.

**Batch Cooking and Meal Prepping Tips:**

- **Prepare Toppings:** Store granola/muesli and raspberries separately to maintain freshness if prepping ahead.
- **Assemble Before Serving:** Assemble the parfaits only when ready to eat to keep the granola crunchy.
- **Portion Control:** Divide Greek yogurt, honey, and granola into single-serving containers to make morning assembly quicker and ensure each serving is balanced.
- **Storage:** Store yogurt and honey together in airtight containers for up to three days to streamline breakfast or snack preparation.

# Scrambled Egg Whites with Bell Peppers and Spinach

- **Preparation Time:** 10 minutes
- **Servings:** 2

Ingredients:

- 4 large egg whites
- 1 cup (150 g) fresh spinach, roughly chopped
- ½ cup (60 g) red bell pepper, diced
- 1 tbsp (15 ml) olive oil
- 1 garlic clove, minced
- ¼ tsp (1.25 ml) paprika
- ¼ tsp (1.25 ml) black pepper

**Nutritional Values (per serving):**

Calories: 90 Protein: 12 g Carbohydrates: 5 g Fat: 2 g Sodium: 90 mg Potassium: 200 mg Phosphorus: 35 mg

**Procedure:**

1. **Prep Ingredients:** Chop the bell pepper into small cubes and roughly chop the spinach.
2. **Whisk Egg Whites:** In a bowl, whisk the egg whites with a pinch of salt and black pepper.
3. **Sauté Vegetables:** In a non-stick skillet, heat olive oil over medium heat. Add minced garlic and diced bell peppers. Cook for 3-4 minutes until the peppers soften.
4. **Add Spinach:** Add the chopped spinach to the skillet and stir until it wilts, about 1-2 minutes.
5. **Scramble Eggs:** Pour the whisked egg whites into the skillet and sprinkle paprika over the mixture. Stir gently with a spatula to combine with the vegetables.
6. **Cook Until Set:** Continue stirring occasionally until the egg whites are fully cooked and no longer translucent, about 3-4 minutes.
7. **Serve Immediately:** Serve the scrambled egg whites with whole-grain toast or a light side salad.

**Batch Cooking and Meal Prepping Tips:**

- **Pre-Chop Ingredients:** Dice bell peppers and chop spinach in advance, storing them separately in airtight containers in the fridge for up to 3 days.
- **Portion Control:** Cook the eggs separately and divide them into single-serving containers. Add vegetables fresh before heating to prevent them from becoming soggy.
- **Storage:** Keep cooked scrambled eggs in the refrigerator for up to two days.

# Smoothie with Blueberries and Low-Potassium Fruits

- **Preparation Time:** 5 minutes
- **Servings:** 2

Ingredients:

- 1 cup (150 g) fresh or frozen blueberries
- ½ cup (80 g) diced pineapple, fresh or frozen
- ½ cup (80 g) diced apple, peeled and cored
- 1 cup (240 ml) unsweetened almond milk
- ½ cup (120 ml) coconut water
- 1 tbsp (15 ml) honey (optional)
- Ice cubes, as needed

**Nutritional Values (per serving):**

Calories: 120 Protein: 2 g Carbohydrates: 26 g Fat: 2 g Sodium: 30 mg Potassium: 120 mg Phosphorus: 30 mg

**Procedure:**

1. **Prepare Ingredients:** Dice the pineapple and apple if using fresh fruit, and measure out the blueberries.
2. **Combine in Blender:** Add all the fruit to a blender, followed by the almond milk and coconut water.
3. **Blend Until Smooth:** Blend on high speed until smooth and creamy. If a thicker consistency is desired, add ice cubes and blend again.
4. **Sweeten (Optional):** If more sweetness is desired, add a tablespoon of honey and blend until combined.
5. **Serve Immediately:** Pour the smoothie into two glasses and serve immediately for a refreshing and nutritious drink.

**Batch Cooking and Meal Prepping Tips:**

- **Prepare Fruit in Advance:** Portion diced fruit into individual freezer bags or airtight containers. When ready to make the smoothie, grab a prepared bag, blend, and go.
- **Freeze Smoothie Packs:** Create "smoothie packs" by combining fruit portions in freezer-safe bags. Add liquids at blending time.
- **Customize:** Use other low-potassium fruits like raspberries or pears to add flavor variations.
- **Storage:** If making multiple servings, pour the extra smoothie into an airtight jar and store it in the fridge for up to 24 hours. Stir or shake well before drinking.

# Quinoa Breakfast Porridge with Apples

- **Preparation Time:** 10 minutes
- **Cooking Time:** 20 minutes
- **Servings:** 2

### Ingredients:

- ½ cup (90 g) quinoa, rinsed
- 1½ cups (360 ml) unsweetened almond milk
- 1 tbsp (15 ml) honey or maple syrup
- 1 tsp (5 ml) ground cinnamon
- 1 apple, cored and diced
- ¼ cup (30 g) sliced almonds or pumpkin seeds
- 1 tbsp (15 ml) chia seeds (optional)

### Nutritional Values (per serving):

Calories: 220 Protein: 7 g Carbohydrates: 32 g Fat: 7 g Sodium: 40 mg Potassium: 180 mg Phosphorus: 90 mg

### Procedure:

1. **Rinse Quinoa:** Place quinoa in a fine-mesh sieve and rinse thoroughly under cold water to remove any bitterness.
2. **Cook Quinoa:** In a medium saucepan, bring the almond milk to a gentle simmer. Add the rinsed quinoa and cook on medium-low heat for about 15-20 minutes until the quinoa is tender and has absorbed most of the liquid.
3. **Flavor Base:** Stir in honey or maple syrup and ground cinnamon. Continue to cook for another 2 minutes, allowing the flavors to meld together.
4. **Prepare Toppings:** While the quinoa cooks, dice the apple into bite-sized cubes.
5. **Serve Porridge:** Divide the quinoa porridge into two bowls. Top with diced apple, sliced almonds or pumpkin seeds, and chia seeds if desired.
6. **Finish & Enjoy:** Add extra almond milk if a looser consistency is desired and serve immediately.

### Batch Cooking and Meal Prepping Tips:

- **Pre-Cook Quinoa:** Cook a larger batch of quinoa ahead of time and store it in the refrigerator for up to 3 days. Reheat portions in almond milk for quick breakfasts.
- **Portion Toppings:** Divide sliced almonds, apples, and chia seeds into small containers for grab-and-go breakfasts.
- **Freeze Portions:** Make extra porridge, portion it into single-serving containers, and freeze. Reheat in the microwave or on the stove.

# Whole Wheat Toast with Low-Potassium Vegetables and Herbs

- **Preparation Time:** 10 minutes
- **Servings:** 2

**Ingredients:**

- 4 slices whole wheat bread
- 1 tbsp (15 ml) olive oil or unsalted butter
- 1 medium zucchini, diced
- ½ cup (60 g) bell peppers, diced
- ¼ cup (30 g) diced cucumber
- 1 tsp (5 ml) dried oregano
- 1 tsp (5 ml) dried thyme
- ¼ tsp (1.25 ml) black pepper
- Pinch of salt (if allowed)
- 2 tbsp (30 g) cream cheese (optional)
- 1 tbsp (15 ml) chopped fresh parsley or cilantro

**Nutritional Values (per serving):**

Calories: 150 Protein: 6 g Carbohydrates: 25 g Fat: 5 g Sodium: 60 mg Potassium: 140 mg Phosphorus: 40 mg

**Procedure:**

1. **Toast Bread:** Toast the whole wheat bread slices until golden brown. Spread a thin layer of cream cheese if using.
2. **Sauté Vegetables:** In a medium skillet, heat olive oil or unsalted butter over medium heat. Add the diced zucchini and bell peppers and sauté for 5-6 minutes until tender. Add the diced cucumber in the last minute to keep it crisp.
3. **Season & Mix:** Add oregano, thyme, black pepper, and a pinch of salt to the sautéed vegetables. Mix well and remove from heat.
4. **Assemble Toast:** Spoon the sautéed vegetable mixture evenly over the toasted bread slices.
5. **Garnish & Serve:** Sprinkle chopped parsley or cilantro over the top before serving.

**Batch Cooking and Meal Prepping Tips:**

- **Pre-Chop Vegetables:** Dice the zucchini and bell peppers in advance and store them in the refrigerator for up to three days for quick preparation.
- **Make Extra Veggie Mix:** Cook extra vegetable topping and store in an airtight container in the refrigerator. Use this as a versatile topping for other dishes like quinoa bowls or scrambled eggs.

# Egg White Omelet with Mushrooms and Chives

- **Preparation Time:** 10 minutes
- **Cooking Time:** 5 minutes
- **Servings:** 2

## Ingredients:

- 6 large egg whites
- 1 cup (100 g) mushrooms, sliced
- 1 tbsp (15 ml) olive oil or unsalted butter
- 2 tbsp (30 ml) fresh chives, chopped
- ¼ tsp (1.25 ml) black pepper
- Pinch of salt (if allowed)

## Nutritional Values (per serving):

Calories: 80 Protein: 10 g Carbohydrates: 3 g Fat: 4 g Sodium: 55 mg Potassium: 160 mg Phosphorus: 35 mg

## Procedure:

1. **Prep Ingredients:** Chop the mushrooms and chives, and separate the egg whites.
2. **Cook Mushrooms:** In a non-stick skillet, heat olive oil or butter over medium heat. Add the sliced mushrooms and cook for 3-4 minutes until softened and slightly browned. Remove from the skillet and set aside.
3. **Whisk Egg Whites:** In a bowl, whisk the egg whites with salt and black pepper.
4. **Pour & Cook:** In the same skillet over medium heat, pour the egg whites and tilt the pan to spread them evenly. Let them cook undisturbed for 2-3 minutes or until set.
5. **Add Filling:** Once the egg whites are mostly set, add the cooked mushrooms and chives to one side of the omelet.
6. **Fold & Finish:** Carefully fold the omelet in half over the filling. Cook for another minute to heat through, then slide the omelet onto a plate.
7. **Serve Immediately:** Garnish with extra chopped chives and serve warm.

## Batch Cooking and Meal Prepping Tips:

- **Pre-Chop Vegetables:** Chop the mushrooms and chives in advance, storing them separately in airtight containers in the fridge for quick assembly.
- **Cook Extra Mushrooms:** Sauté extra mushrooms to use as a filling in other breakfast items like scrambled eggs or toast throughout the week.
- **Store Omelets:** Make a few omelets ahead of time and store them in individual containers in the fridge for up to 2 days. Reheat gently on the stovetop or microwave before eating.

# Cottage Cheese with Low-Potassium Fruit

- **Preparation Time:** 5 minutes
- **Servings:** 2

Ingredients:

- 1 cup (240 g) low-fat cottage cheese
- ½ cup (75 g) diced strawberries
- ½ cup (75 g) diced blueberries
- ½ cup (75 g) diced pears
- 2 tbsp (30 ml) honey or maple syrup
- 2 tbsp (30 g) sliced almonds or pumpkin seeds

**Nutritional Values (per serving):**

Calories: 150 Protein: 10 g Carbohydrates: 22 g Fat: 4 g Sodium: 400 mg Potassium: 180 mg Phosphorus: 110 mg

**Procedure:**

1. **Prepare Fruits:** Dice the strawberries, blueberries, and pears. Set aside in a small bowl.
2. **Assemble Base:** Divide the cottage cheese evenly into two bowls or cups.
3. **Top with Fruit:** Add the diced fruits on top of the cottage cheese, spreading them evenly between both servings.
4. **Sweeten:** Drizzle honey or maple syrup over each serving for sweetness.
5. **Add Nuts/Seeds:** Sprinkle sliced almonds or pumpkin seeds on top for added crunch.
6. **Serve Immediately:** Enjoy as a quick breakfast or snack, or cover and refrigerate for later.

**Batch Cooking and Meal Prepping Tips:**

- **Pre-Chop Fruit:** Dice the fruits ahead of time and store them in individual airtight containers in the refrigerator.
- **Prepare Cottage Cheese Base:** Divide the cottage cheese into multiple portion-sized containers in advance.
- **Mix and Store:** Layer the ingredients (cottage cheese, fruit, honey, and nuts/seeds) in jars for easy grab-and-go snacks or breakfast options.
- **Storage:** Store pre-assembled parfaits in the refrigerator for up to 2 days. Give them a gentle stir before serving to mix the flavors.

# Warm Millet Cereal with Almond Milk and Strawberries

- **Preparation Time:** 5 minutes
- **Cooking Time:** 20 minutes
- **Servings:** 2

### Ingredients:

- ½ cup (90 g) millet, rinsed
- 2 cups (480 ml) unsweetened almond milk
- 1 tbsp (15 ml) honey or maple syrup
- 1 tsp (5 ml) ground cinnamon
- ½ tsp (2.5 ml) vanilla extract
- 1 cup (150 g) fresh strawberries, hulled and sliced
- 2 tbsp (30 g) sliced almonds or pumpkin seeds

### Nutritional Values (per serving):

Calories: 200 Protein: 5 g Carbohydrates: 35 g Fat: 6 g Sodium: 80 mg Potassium: 150 mg Phosphorus: 90 mg

### Procedure:

1. **Rinse Millet:** Rinse the millet thoroughly in a fine-mesh sieve under cold water.
2. **Simmer Millet:** In a medium saucepan, bring the almond milk to a gentle simmer. Add the rinsed millet, reduce heat to medium-low, and simmer for 15-20 minutes until the millet is tender and has absorbed most of the liquid. Stir occasionally.
3. **Flavor Base:** Stir in the honey or maple syrup, cinnamon, and vanilla extract. Mix well to distribute the flavors.
4. **Prepare Strawberries:** While the millet simmers, hull and slice the strawberries. **Serve Cereal:** Divide the millet cereal into two bowls. Top with the sliced strawberries and sprinkle sliced almonds or pumpkin seeds on top.
5. **Finish & Enjoy:** Add extra almond milk if a looser consistency is desired, and serve immediately while warm.

### Batch Cooking and Meal Prepping Tips:

- **Pre-Cook Millet:** Cook extra millet in almond milk, and store it in an airtight container in the fridge for up to 3 days. Reheat portions with extra almond milk for quick breakfast.
- **Pre-Cut Strawberries:** Slice strawberries and keep them in a separate airtight container for easy assembly in the morning.
- **Mix Ahead:** Combine all the dry ingredients (millet, spices, seeds) in advance to save prep time. Add liquid and cook when ready.

# Whole Wheat English Muffin with Almond Butter

- **Preparation Time:** 5 minutes
- **Servings:** 2

**Ingredients:**

- 2 whole wheat English muffins, split
- 2 tbsp (30 ml) almond butter
- 1 tsp (5 ml) honey (optional)
- 2 tbsp (30 g) sliced almonds

**Nutritional Values (per serving):**

Calories: 190 Protein: 7 g Carbohydrates: 25 g Fat: 7 g Sodium: 180 mg Potassium: 150 mg Phosphorus: 60 mg

**Procedure:**

1. **Toast Muffins:** Split the whole wheat English muffins and toast until golden brown.
2. **Spread Almond Butter:** Evenly spread 1 tbsp (15 ml) of almond butter on each toasted English muffin half.
3. **Drizzle Honey:** Add a light drizzle of honey over the almond butter, if desired, for added sweetness.
4. **Top with Almonds:** Sprinkle sliced almonds on top for added crunch and flavor.
5. **Serve Immediately:** Serve warm as a quick breakfast or snack.

**Batch Cooking and Meal Prepping Tips:**

- **Pre-Slice Muffins:** Slice the English muffins ahead of time to make toasting faster. Store in an airtight bag or container.
- **Portion Almond Butter:** Divide almond butter into small containers for easy spreading in the morning.
- **Storage:** Pre-toast muffins and store them in the refrigerator for up to 2 days. Warm them gently in a toaster oven or skillet before serving.
- **Portable Option:** Assemble ahead of time and wrap the English muffin halves for on-the-go breakfasts.

# Buckwheat Pancakes with Fresh Fruit

- **Preparation Time:** 10 minutes
- **Cooking Time:** 15 minutes
- **Servings:** 4

## Ingredients:

- 1 cup (120 g) buckwheat flour
- 1 tbsp (15 ml) honey or maple syrup
- 1 tsp (5 ml) baking powder
- ½ tsp (2.5 ml) baking soda
- 1 tsp (5 ml) ground cinnamon
- 1 cup (240 ml) unsweetened almond milk
- 2 large egg whites
- 1 tsp (5 ml) vanilla extract
- 1 tbsp (15 ml) olive oil or melted coconut oil
- 1 cup (150 g) fresh fruit, such as blueberries, strawberries, or raspberries

## Nutritional Values (per serving):

Calories: 140 Protein: 5 g Carbohydrates: 30 g Fat: 2 g Sodium: 120 mg Potassium: 160 mg Phosphorus: 80 mg

## Procedure:

1. **Prepare Dry Ingredients:** In a large mixing bowl, combine the buckwheat flour, baking powder, baking soda, and cinnamon. Mix well.
2. **Whisk Wet Ingredients:** In another bowl, whisk together the almond milk, egg whites, honey or maple syrup, vanilla extract, and olive oil or melted coconut oil.
3. **Combine Wet and Dry:** Pour the wet ingredients into the bowl with the dry ingredients and stir until just combined. Do not overmix, as some lumps are fine.
4. **Preheat & Grease Pan:** Preheat a non-stick skillet or griddle over medium heat. Lightly grease with olive oil or cooking spray. **Cook Pancakes:** Pour ¼ cup (60 ml) of batter onto the skillet for each pancake. Cook for 2-3 minutes until bubbles form on the surface, then flip and cook for another 1-2 minutes until golden brown. Repeat with the remaining batter.
5. **Top with Fruit:** Serve the pancakes warm, topped with fresh fruit of your choice.

## Batch Cooking and Meal Prepping Tips:

- **Pre-Make Pancake Mix:** Combine dry ingredients in a jar to create a pancake mix that only requires adding wet ingredients when ready to cook.
- **Fruit Preparation:** Wash and slice the fruit ahead of time.

# Poached Egg Whites over Arugula and Roasted Red Peppers

- **Preparation Time:** 10 minutes
- **Cooking Time:** 5 minutes
- **Servings:** 2

## Ingredients:

- 4 large egg whites
- 2 cups (60 g) fresh arugula, washed and dried
- ½ cup (60 g) roasted red peppers, thinly sliced
- 1 tbsp (15 ml) olive oil
- 1 tbsp (15 ml) lemon juice
- ¼ tsp (1.25 ml) black pepper
- Pinch of salt (if allowed)
- Fresh herbs, like parsley or basil, for garnish

## Nutritional Values (per serving):

Calories: 80 Protein: 9 g Carbohydrates: 4 g Fat: 4 g Sodium: 120 mg Potassium: 160 mg Phosphorus: 50 mg

## Procedure:

1. **Prep Vegetables:** Wash and dry the arugula and slice the roasted red peppers.
2. **Season Arugula:** In a bowl, toss the arugula with olive oil, lemon juice, black pepper, and salt (if desired). Divide between two serving plates.
3. **Poach Egg Whites:**
   - Bring a pot of water to a gentle simmer.
   - Crack the egg whites into separate small bowls.
   - Create a gentle whirlpool in the water using a spoon and slide each bowl of egg whites into the center.
   - Poach for about 3-4 minutes, or until the whites are set but still soft. Remove the poached whites carefully with a slotted spoon and drain excess water.
4. **Assemble Plate:** Place the poached egg whites on top of the arugula, then add a portion of the roasted red peppers around each.
5. **Garnish & Serve:** Garnish with fresh herbs like parsley or basil for extra flavor. Serve immediately.

## Batch Cooking and Meal Prepping Tips:

- **Pre-Wash Arugula:** Rinse and dry the arugula in advance, storing it in an airtight container with a paper towel to absorb excess moisture.
- **Poach Ahead:** Poach egg whites in advance and store them in cold water in the fridge. Reheat gently in simmering water before serving.

# Tofu Scramble with Turmeric and Diced Zucchini

- **Preparation Time:** 10 minutes
- **Cooking Time:** 10 minutes
- **Servings:** 2

Ingredients:

- 1 package (14 oz or 400 g) firm tofu, drained
- 1 tbsp (15 ml) olive oil
- 1 medium zucchini, diced
- ½ tsp (2.5 ml) turmeric powder
- ¼ tsp (1.25 ml) cumin powder
- ¼ tsp (1.25 ml) black pepper
- Pinch of salt (if permitted)
- 2 tbsp (30 ml) nutritional yeast
- 2 tbsp (30 g) chopped fresh parsley or cilantro

**Nutritional Values (per serving):**

Calories: 180 Protein: 12 g Carbohydrates: 8 g Fat: 10 g Sodium: 70 mg Potassium: 160 mg Phosphorus: 90 mg

**Procedure:**

1. **Prep Tofu:** Drain the tofu and crumble it with your hands or a fork into small chunks resembling scrambled eggs.
2. **Cook Zucchini:** In a large skillet, heat olive oil over medium heat. Add diced zucchini and sauté for 4-5 minutes until softened. **Add Tofu:** Add crumbled tofu to the skillet, stirring to combine with the zucchini.
3. **Season & Cook:** Sprinkle turmeric, cumin, black pepper, and salt over the mixture. Stir well and cook for another 3-4 minutes until the tofu is heated through and evenly colored.
4. **Enhance Flavor:** Stir in the nutritional yeast and cook for 1-2 minutes longer, allowing the flavors to meld together.
5. **Garnish & Serve:** Garnish with chopped fresh parsley or cilantro. Serve immediately as a standalone dish or with whole wheat toast.

**Batch Cooking and Meal Prepping Tips:**

- **Prep Tofu in Advance:** Drain and crumble the tofu ahead of time, storing it in an airtight container in the fridge for up to 2 days.
- **Pre-Cut Zucchini:** Dice the zucchini and store it in an airtight container to save time during cooking.
- **Large Batch Cooking:** Make a larger batch and store individual portions in the fridge for up to 3 days. Reheat gently in a skillet or microwave.

# Berry Smoothie with Spinach and Flaxseed

- **Preparation Time:** 5 minutes
- **Servings:** 2

Ingredients:

- 1 cup (150 g) mixed berries (blueberries, strawberries, raspberries), fresh or frozen
- 1 cup (30 g) fresh spinach, washed
- 1 tbsp (15 ml) ground flaxseed
- 1 cup (240 ml) unsweetened almond milk
- ½ cup (120 ml) coconut water
- 1 tbsp (15 ml) honey or maple syrup (optional)
- Ice cubes, as needed

Nutritional Values (per serving):

Calories: 120 Protein: 3 g Carbohydrates: 20 g Fat: 3 g Sodium: 50 mg Potassium: 180 mg Phosphorus: 40 mg

Procedure:

1. **Combine Ingredients:** Add the mixed berries, spinach, ground flaxseed, almond milk, coconut water, and honey (if using) to a blender.
2. **Blend Until Smooth:** Blend on high speed until smooth and creamy. If a thicker consistency is desired, add ice cubes and blend again.
3. **Serve Immediately:** Pour the smoothie into two glasses and enjoy as a refreshing, nutrient-packed breakfast or snack.

Batch Cooking and Meal Prepping Tips:

- **Portion Fruit:** Pre-portion mixed berries and spinach into separate freezer bags or airtight containers for quick access.
- **Customize Flavor:** Adjust the fruit or add other low-potassium fruits like pears or apples for variety.
- **Smoothie Packs:** Create "smoothie packs" by adding pre-measured fruit and spinach into freezer bags. Add liquids at blending time for a quicker process.
- **Storage:** Make extra smoothies and store them in airtight containers in the fridge for up to 24 hours. Shake well before drinking.

# Sweet Potato Hash

- **Preparation Time:** 10 minutes
- **Cooking Time:** 15 minutes
- **Servings:** 2

### Ingredients:

- 1 large sweet potato, peeled and diced (about 2 cups or 300 g)
- 1 tbsp (15 ml) olive oil
- 1 medium onion, diced
- 1 red bell pepper, diced
- 1 tsp (5 ml) smoked paprika
- ½ tsp (2.5 ml) cumin powder
- ¼ tsp (1.25 ml) black pepper
- Pinch of salt (if allowed)
- 2 tbsp (30 g) chopped fresh parsley or cilantro

### Nutritional Values (per serving):

Calories: 140 Protein: 3 g Carbohydrates: 27 g Fat: 4 g Sodium: 55 mg Potassium: 350 mg Phosphorus: 50 mg

### Procedure:

1. **Prep Vegetables:** Peel and dice the sweet potato, onion, and bell pepper into bite-sized cubes.
2. **Cook Sweet Potato:** In a large skillet, heat olive oil over medium-high heat. Add diced sweet potatoes and cook for 8-10 minutes, stirring occasionally, until the potatoes begin to soften and develop a golden-brown crust.
3. **Add Onion & Pepper:** Add diced onion and bell pepper to the skillet. Cook for another 5-7 minutes until the vegetables are tender.
4. **Season & Stir:** Add smoked paprika, cumin powder, black pepper, and a pinch of salt. Stir well to coat the vegetables evenly with the spices.
5. **Garnish & Serve:** Remove from heat and garnish with chopped parsley or cilantro. Serve hot as a hearty breakfast or brunch dish.

### Batch Cooking and Meal Prepping Tips:

- **Pre-Cut Vegetables:** Dice sweet potatoes, onions, and bell peppers ahead of time and store them in airtight containers for up to 2 days.
- **Batch Cooking:** Prepare a larger batch and store individual portions in airtight containers in the refrigerator for up to 3 days. Reheat gently in a skillet or microwave before serving.
- **Enhance Flavor:** Customize the dish with additional spices like thyme or oregano, or by adding low-potassium vegetables like zucchini or mushrooms.

# Oat Bran Muffins

- **Preparation Time:** 10 minutes
- **Cooking Time:** 15-18 minutes
- **Servings:** 12 muffins

### Ingredients:

- 1 cup (120 g) oat bran
- 1 cup (120 g) whole wheat flour
- 1 tsp (5 ml) baking powder
- ½ tsp (2.5 ml) baking soda
- ½ tsp (2.5 ml) cinnamon
- ¼ tsp (1.25 ml) salt (optional)
- 1 cup (240 ml) unsweetened applesauce
- ½ cup (120 ml) unsweetened almond milk
- ¼ cup (60 ml) honey or maple syrup
- 2 large egg whites
- 2 tbsp (30 ml) olive oil or melted coconut oil
- 1 tsp (5 ml) vanilla extract
- ½ cup (75 g) fresh or frozen berries (optional)

### Nutritional Values (per muffin):

Calories: 110 Protein: 4 g Carbohydrates: 20 g Fat: 3 g Sodium: 80 mg Potassium: 150 mg Phosphorus: 60 mg

### Procedure:

1. **Preheat Oven:** Preheat the oven to 375°F (190°C). Line a muffin tin with paper liners or lightly grease with oil.
2. **Combine Dry Ingredients:** In a large mixing bowl, mix oat bran, whole wheat flour, baking powder, baking soda, cinnamon, and salt (if using).
3. **Whisk Wet Ingredients:** In a separate bowl, whisk together applesauce, almond milk, honey or maple syrup, egg whites, olive oil, and vanilla extract until well combined.
4. **Combine Wet & Dry:** Pour the wet ingredients into the dry ingredients and mix gently until just combined. If using berries, fold them into the batter.
5. **Fill Muffin Tin:** Divide the batter evenly among the muffin cups, filling each about ¾ full.
6. **Bake:** Bake in the preheated oven for 15-18 minutes, or until a toothpick inserted into the center comes out clean.
7. **Cool & Serve:** Let the muffins cool in the tin for 5 minutes before transferring them to a wire rack to cool completely.

# Polenta with Low-Potassium Mushrooms and Herbs

- **Preparation Time:** 10 minutes
- **Cooking Time:** 20 minutes
- **Servings:** 2

## Ingredients:

- 1 cup (240 ml) water
- 1 cup (240 ml) unsweetened almond milk
- ½ cup (80 g) polenta or coarse cornmeal
- 1 tbsp (15 ml) olive oil or unsalted butter
- 1 cup (150 g) oyster or shiitake mushrooms, sliced
- ½ cup (75 g) diced zucchini
- 1 garlic clove, minced
- ½ tsp (2.5 ml) dried thyme
- ¼ tsp (1.25 ml) black pepper
- Pinch of salt (if allowed)
- 2 tbsp (30 ml) fresh parsley or basil, chopped

**Nutritional Values (per serving):**

Calories: 150 Protein: 4 g Carbohydrates: 25 g Fat: 4 g Sodium: 30 mg Potassium: 180 mg Phosphorus: 50 mg

## Procedure:

1. **Cook Polenta:** In a medium saucepan, bring the water and almond milk to a gentle boil. Slowly add the polenta while stirring continuously to prevent lumps. Reduce heat to low and cook for 15-20 minutes, stirring frequently until the polenta thickens.

2. **Sauté Mushrooms and Vegetables:**
   - In a skillet, heat olive oil or butter over medium heat.
   - Add the sliced mushrooms, zucchini, and minced garlic. Sauté for 5-7 minutes until the vegetables are tender.

3. **Season:** Add dried thyme, black pepper, and a pinch of salt (if using). Stir well to combine the flavors and cook for another minute.

4. **Serve Polenta:** Divide the cooked polenta between two bowls and top with the sautéed mushrooms and vegetables. **Garnish:** Sprinkle with fresh parsley or basil for added flavor. Serve immediately while warm.

## Batch Cooking and Meal Prepping Tips:

- **Pre-Cut Vegetables:** Dice zucchini and slice mushrooms in advance, storing them in airtight containers in the fridge for up to 2 days. **Pre-Cook Polenta:** Make a larger batch of polenta, let it cool, and slice it into squares. Store in the fridge and reheat by sautéing or microwaving.

# Farina Porridge with Peaches

- **Preparation Time:** 5 minutes
- **Cooking Time:** 10 minutes
- **Servings:** 2

## Ingredients:

- 2 cups (480 ml) unsweetened almond milk
- ½ cup (80 g) farina (cream of wheat)
- 1 tbsp (15 ml) honey or maple syrup
- ½ tsp (2.5 ml) ground cinnamon
- 1 tsp (5 ml) vanilla extract
- 1 cup (150 g) fresh or canned peaches, diced (low-sugar if canned)

## Nutritional Values (per serving):

Calories: 170 Protein: 5 g Carbohydrates: 30 g Fat: 3 g Sodium: 35 mg Potassium: 120 mg Phosphorus: 50 mg

## Procedure:

1. **Boil Almond Milk:** In a medium saucepan, bring the almond milk to a gentle boil over medium heat.
2. **Add Farina:** Gradually add the farina to the boiling milk while stirring continuously to prevent lumps.
3. **Cook Until Thickened:** Reduce the heat to low and cook for about 5-7 minutes, stirring frequently until the mixture thickens to a porridge consistency.
4. **Flavor Base:** Stir in honey or maple syrup, cinnamon, and vanilla extract. Mix well to distribute the flavors evenly.
5. **Top with Peaches:** Divide the porridge into two bowls and top with diced peaches.
6. **Serve Immediately:** Add extra almond milk if a looser consistency is desired. Serve warm while garnished with additional cinnamon if desired.

## Batch Cooking and Meal Prepping Tips:

- **Pre-Cut Peaches:** Dice fresh or canned peaches in advance and store them in an airtight container in the fridge for up to 2 days.
- **Pre-Mix Dry Ingredients:** Combine farina, cinnamon, and vanilla extract in a jar to save time during preparation.
- **Cook Larger Batches:** Cook extra portions of porridge and store them in the fridge for up to 2 days. Reheat gently in the microwave or on the stove with extra almond milk.

# Whole Grain Waffles with Coconut Yogurt

- **Preparation Time:** 10 minutes
- **Cooking Time:** 15 minutes
- **Servings:** 4

**Ingredients:**

- 1 cup (120 g) whole wheat flour
- ½ cup (60 g) oat flour (or finely ground rolled oats)
- 1 tsp (5 ml) baking powder
- ½ tsp (2.5 ml) baking soda
- 1 tsp (5 ml) ground cinnamon
- ¼ tsp (1.25 ml) salt (optional)
- 1 cup (240 ml) unsweetened almond milk
- 2 large egg whites
- 2 tbsp (30 ml) olive oil or melted coconut oil
- 1 tsp (5 ml) vanilla extract
- 1 cup (240 ml) coconut yogurt
- Fresh fruit, like strawberries, for topping

**Nutritional Values (per serving):**

Calories: 180 Protein: 6 g Carbohydrates: 28 g Fat: 6 g Sodium: 85 mg Potassium: 150 mg Phosphorus: 60 mg

**Procedure:**

1. **Preheat Waffle Iron:** Preheat your waffle iron according to the manufacturer's instructions.
2. **Mix Dry Ingredients:** In a large mixing bowl, combine whole wheat flour, oat flour, baking powder, baking soda, cinnamon, and salt. Mix well.
3. **Whisk Wet Ingredients:** In a separate bowl, whisk together almond milk, egg whites, olive oil or melted coconut oil, and vanilla extract until smooth. **Combine Wet & Dry:** Pour the wet ingredients into the dry ingredients and stir gently until just combined. Do not overmix; some lumps are okay.
4. **Cook Waffles:** Lightly grease the waffle iron and pour enough batter to fill it. Cook for 3-4 minutes or until the waffles are golden brown and crisp. Repeat with remaining batter.
5. **Serve with Yogurt:** Serve the waffles warm, topped with a dollop of coconut yogurt and your favorite fresh fruit.

**Batch Cooking and Meal Prepping Tips:**

- **Pre-Mix Dry Ingredients:** Combine the dry ingredients in a jar to have a ready-to-go waffle mix. Just add wet ingredients and cook when ready. **Cook Extra & Freeze:** Cook extra waffles and freeze them in a single layer. Once frozen, transfer to a resealable bag. Reheat in a toaster for a quick breakfast.

# Rice Cakes Topped with Hummus and Herbs

- **Preparation Time:** 5 minutes
- **Servings:** 2

Ingredients:

- 4 plain or whole-grain rice cakes
- ½ cup (120 g) hummus
- 1 tbsp (15 ml) lemon juice
- 1 tsp (5 ml) ground cumin
- ¼ tsp (1.25 ml) black pepper
- Pinch of salt (if allowed)
- 2 tbsp (30 g) fresh parsley or cilantro, chopped
- 1 tbsp (15 ml) olive oil (optional)

**Nutritional Values (per serving):**

Calories: 110 Protein: 3 g Carbohydrates: 20 g Fat: 3 g Sodium: 80 mg Potassium: 100 mg Phosphorus: 40 mg

**Procedure:**

1. **Prepare Hummus:** In a small bowl, combine hummus, lemon juice, cumin, black pepper, and salt (if allowed). Mix well.
2. **Assemble Rice Cakes:** Spread a generous amount of the seasoned hummus on each rice cake.
3. **Garnish & Drizzle:** Top with chopped parsley or cilantro and drizzle with olive oil, if desired.
4. **Serve Immediately:** Serve the rice cakes as a quick breakfast, snack, or light meal.

**Batch Cooking and Meal Prepping Tips:**

- **Season Ahead:** Mix lemon juice, cumin, and other seasonings into a larger batch of hummus and store in the fridge for up to 3 days.
- **Pre-Chop Herbs:** Chop parsley or cilantro in advance and keep it in an airtight container for quicker assembly.
- **Assemble Before Eating:** Keep rice cakes and hummus separate until just before serving to prevent them from becoming soggy.

# Lunch

## Quinoa Salad with Roasted Low-Potassium Vegetables

- **Preparation Time:** 15 minutes
- **Cooking Time:** 30 minutes
- **Servings:** 4

### Ingredients:

- 1 cup (170 g) quinoa, rinsed
- 2 cups (480 ml) water or low-sodium vegetable broth
- 1 medium zucchini, diced
- 1 red bell pepper, diced
- 1 small eggplant, diced
- 1 tbsp (15 ml) olive oil
- ½ tsp (2.5 ml) paprika
- ½ tsp (2.5 ml) dried thyme
- ¼ tsp (1.25 ml) black pepper
- Pinch of salt (if permitted)
- 1 tbsp (15 ml) lemon juice
- 1 tsp (5 ml) Dijon mustard
- 2 tbsp (30 g) fresh parsley or cilantro, chopped

### Nutritional Values (per serving):

Calories: 160 Protein: 5 g Carbohydrates: 26 g Fat: 5 g Sodium: 50 mg Potassium: 200 mg Phosphorus: 60 mg

### Procedure:

1. **Cook Quinoa:** In a medium saucepan, bring the water or broth to a boil. Add the rinsed quinoa, reduce heat, cover, and simmer for 15 minutes until tender. Remove from heat and let it sit for 5 minutes, then fluff with a fork.
2. **Roast Vegetables:** Preheat the oven to 400°F (200°C). On a baking sheet, toss zucchini, bell pepper, and eggplant with olive oil, paprika, thyme, black pepper, and salt (if permitted). Spread in an even layer and roast for 20-25 minutes until tender and lightly browned.
3. **Make Dressing:** In a small bowl, whisk together lemon juice, Dijon mustard, and olive oil.
4. **Combine Salad:** In a large mixing bowl, combine the cooked quinoa with the roasted vegetables. Add the dressing and mix well.
5. **Garnish & Serve:** Garnish with fresh parsley or cilantro and serve the salad warm or chilled.

### Batch Cooking and Meal Prepping Tips:

- **Pre-Roast Vegetables:** Roast a bigger batch of vegetables to use in other meals, such as wraps or pasta.

# Lentil Soup

- **Preparation Time:** 10 minutes
- **Cooking Time:** 30-35 minutes
- **Servings:** 4

### Ingredients:

- 1 cup (190 g) dried green or brown lentils, rinsed and drained
- 1 tbsp (15 ml) olive oil
- 1 medium onion, diced
- 2 medium carrots, diced
- 2 celery stalks, diced
- 2 garlic cloves, minced
- 1 tsp (5 ml) ground cumin
- ½ tsp (2.5 ml) ground coriander
- ½ tsp (2.5 ml) paprika
- ¼ tsp (1.25 ml) black pepper
- Pinch of salt (if allowed)
- 6 cups (1.5 L) low-sodium vegetable broth or water
- 2 tbsp (30 g) tomato paste
- 1 bay leaf
- 1 tbsp (15 ml) lemon juice
- 2 tbsp (30 g) chopped fresh parsley or cilantro

### Nutritional Values (per serving):

Calories: 180 Protein: 10 g Carbohydrates: 30 g Fat: 4 g Sodium: 50 mg Potassium: 250 mg Phosphorus: 80 mg

### Procedure:

1. **Prep Vegetables:** Dice the onion, carrots, and celery, and mince the garlic.
2. **Sauté Vegetables:** In a large pot, heat the olive oil over medium heat. Add the diced onion, carrots, and celery. Sauté for about 5 minutes until softened, then add the garlic and spices (cumin, coriander, paprika, black pepper, and salt). Cook for another 1-2 minutes until fragrant.
3. **Add Lentils & Broth:** Add the rinsed lentils, vegetable broth or water, tomato paste, and bay leaf. Stir to combine.
4. **Simmer:** Bring to a boil, then reduce the heat to low and cover. Simmer for 30-35 minutes or until the lentils are tender.
5. **Finish:** Remove the bay leaf and stir in the lemon juice and fresh parsley or cilantro. Adjust seasoning as needed. **Serve:** Ladle the soup into bowls and serve warm.

### Batch Cooking and Meal Prepping Tips:

- **Make Extra:** Prepare a larger batch and store in airtight containers in the fridge for up to 3 days or freeze for up to 3 months.
- **Portion Control:** Divide into individual servings for easy grab-and-go meals.

# Grilled Chicken Wrap with Lettuce and Tomato

- **Preparation Time:** 10 minutes
- **Cooking Time:** 10 minutes
- **Servings:** 2

### Ingredients:

- 1 medium chicken breast (about 8 oz or 225 g)
- 1 tbsp (15 ml) olive oil
- 1 tsp (5 ml) lemon juice
- ½ tsp (2.5 ml) paprika
- ¼ tsp (1.25 ml) black pepper
- Pinch of salt (if allowed)
- 2 large whole wheat tortillas
- 2-3 leaves of romaine or iceberg lettuce
- 1 medium tomato, sliced
- 2 tbsp (30 ml) hummus or low-fat yogurt dressing
- 2 tbsp (30 g) shredded cheese (optional)

### Nutritional Values (per serving):

Calories: 230 Protein: 15 g Carbohydrates: 20 g Fat: 8 g Sodium: 90 mg Potassium: 180 mg Phosphorus: 90 mg

### Procedure:

1. **Prepare Chicken Marinade:** In a small bowl, combine olive oil, lemon juice, paprika, black pepper, and salt (if using).
2. **Marinate Chicken:** Rub the marinade over the chicken breast and let it sit for 10 minutes.
3. **Grill Chicken:** Preheat a grill or grill pan over medium heat. Grill the chicken breast for 5-6 minutes on each side or until fully cooked and the internal temperature reaches 165°F (74°C). Let it rest for 5 minutes, then slice into thin strips.
4. **Assemble Wraps:**
   - Warm the tortillas briefly on the grill or in a dry skillet.
   - Spread 1 tbsp of hummus or low-fat dressing on each tortilla.
   - Add lettuce leaves, tomato slices, and shredded cheese if desired.
   - Place the sliced chicken breast on top and wrap tightly.
5. **Serve:** Cut each wrap in half and serve immediately with a side salad or fresh fruit.

### Batch Cooking and Meal Prepping Tips:

- **Wrap Before Eating:** To avoid sogginess, wrap just before eating or pack ingredients separately for meal prep.

# Egg White Salad Sandwich on Whole Grain Bread

- **Preparation Time:** 15 minutes
- **Cooking Time:** 10 minutes
- **Servings:** 2

Ingredients:

- 6 large egg whites
- 1 tbsp (15 ml) plain Greek yogurt or low-fat mayonnaise
- 1 tsp (5 ml) Dijon mustard
- 1 tsp (5 ml) lemon juice
- ½ tsp (2.5 ml) black pepper
- Pinch of salt (if allowed)
- 2 tbsp (30 g) celery, finely diced
- 1 tbsp (15 g) scallions, finely chopped
- 4 slices whole grain bread
- 2-3 leaves romaine or iceberg lettuce
- 1 medium tomato, sliced

**Nutritional Values (per serving):**

Calories: 180 Protein: 15 g Carbohydrates: 22 g Fat: 3 g Sodium: 160 mg Potassium: 170 mg Phosphorus: 80 mg

**Procedure:**

1. **Boil Egg Whites:** Fill a saucepan with water and bring it to a boil. Add egg whites (or whole eggs if you prefer) and cook for 8-10 minutes until fully set. Drain and transfer to an ice bath to cool. Once cooled, peel the eggs and chop the whites into small pieces.
2. **Mix Dressing:** In a bowl, mix together Greek yogurt or mayonnaise, Dijon mustard, lemon juice, black pepper, and salt (if using).
3. **Combine Salad:** Add the chopped egg whites, diced celery, and scallions to the dressing and mix well to combine. Adjust seasoning to taste.
4. **Assemble Sandwich:**
    - Toast the whole grain bread slices if desired.
    - Place lettuce leaves and tomato slices on one side of the bread.
    - Spread a generous amount of egg white salad over the lettuce and top with another bread slice.
5. **Serve Immediately:** Cut each sandwich in half and serve warm or cold, optionally with a side salad.

# Salmon Salad with Greens

- **Preparation Time:** 10 minutes
- **Cooking Time:** 10 minutes
- **Servings:** 2

### Ingredients:

- 1 salmon fillet (about 8 oz or 225 g)
- 1 tbsp (15 ml) olive oil
- 1 tbsp (15 ml) lemon juice
- ½ tsp (2.5 ml) paprika
- ¼ tsp (1.25 ml) black pepper
- Pinch of salt (if allowed)
- 4 cups (120 g) mixed greens (like spinach, arugula, or kale)
- 1 medium cucumber, sliced
- 1 small carrot, shredded
- 1 medium tomato, diced
- 1 tbsp (15 g) sunflower seeds or pumpkin seeds (optional)

### Dressing:

- 1 tbsp (15 ml) olive oil
- 1 tbsp (15 ml) balsamic vinegar
- 1 tsp (5 ml) Dijon mustard
- 1 tsp (5 ml) honey / maple syrup

### Nutritional Values (per serving):

Calories: 220 Protein: 20 g Carbohydrates: 15 g Fat: 10 g Sodium: 80 mg Potassium: 200 mg Phosphorus: 100 mg

### Procedure:

1. **Season Salmon:** Rub the salmon fillet with olive oil, lemon juice, paprika, black pepper, and salt (if using).
2. **Cook Salmon:** Heat a non-stick skillet over medium heat. Add the salmon fillet, skin side down, and cook for 4-5 minutes per side or until fully cooked. Remove and let it cool slightly, then flake into bite-sized pieces.
3. **Prepare Salad:** In a large bowl, mix the greens with cucumber slices, shredded carrot, and diced tomato.
4. **Mix Dressing:** In a small bowl, whisk together olive oil, balsamic vinegar, Dijon mustard, and honey until emulsified.
5. **Assemble Salad:** Drizzle the dressing over the greens and toss to combine. Divide the salad between two bowls and top with flaked salmon and sunflower or pumpkin seeds.
6. **Serve Immediately:** Serve the salad while the salmon is still warm or chilled, if preferred.

# Chickpea Curry

- **Preparation Time:** 10 minutes
- **Cooking Time:** 20 minutes
- **Servings:** 4

### Ingredients:

- 1 tbsp (15 ml) olive oil or coconut oil
- 1 medium onion, diced
- 2 garlic cloves, minced
- 1 tbsp (15 ml) grated ginger
- 2 tsp (10 ml) curry powder
- 1 tsp (5 ml) ground cumin
- ½ tsp (2.5 ml) paprika
- ¼ tsp (1.25 ml) black pepper
- Pinch of salt (if allowed)
- 2 cups (480 ml) low-sodium vegetable broth
- 1 can (15 oz or 425 g) chickpeas, drained and rinsed
- 1 can (14 oz or 400 ml) diced tomatoes
- 1 cup (240 ml) unsweetened coconut milk
- 1 cup (150 g) diced zucchini
- 2 tbsp (30 g) chopped fresh cilantro or parsley

### Nutritional Values (per serving):

Calories: 180 Protein: 6 g Carbohydrates: 22 g Fat: 8 g Sodium: 90 mg Potassium: 190 mg Phosphorus: 80 mg

### Procedure:

1. **Sauté Aromatics:** In a large pot or skillet, heat the olive oil over medium heat. Add the diced onion and cook for 5 minutes until softened. Stir in the garlic and ginger and sauté for another 1-2 minutes until fragrant.
2. **Add Spices:** Add the curry powder, cumin, paprika, black pepper, and salt (if using). Stir for 1 minute to toast the spices.
3. **Combine Ingredients:** Add the vegetable broth, chickpeas, diced tomatoes, coconut milk, and diced zucchini. Mix well.
4. **Simmer:** Bring to a gentle boil, then reduce the heat to low and let it simmer for 15-20 minutes until the zucchini is tender and the flavors meld together.
5. **Finish & Garnish:** Remove from heat and stir in fresh cilantro or parsley. Adjust seasoning to taste.
6. **Serve:** Ladle the chickpea curry into bowls and serve with steamed rice, naan, or as a standalone dish.

**Batch Cooking and Meal Prepping Tips: Portion Control:** Divide the curry into individual servings for grab-and-go lunches or dinners.

# Roasted Turkey Sandwich with Cucumber and Mustard

- **Preparation Time:** 10 minutes
- **Servings:** 2

### Ingredients:

- 4 slices whole grain bread
- 4 oz (115 g) roasted turkey breast, sliced thinly
- 1 medium cucumber, thinly sliced
- 2 tbsp (30 ml) Dijon mustard
- 2-3 leaves romaine or iceberg lettuce
- 2 tbsp (30 g) shredded carrots
- 1 tsp (5 ml) lemon juice
- ¼ tsp (1.25 ml) black pepper
- Pinch of salt (if allowed)

### Nutritional Values (per serving):

Calories: 200 Protein: 15 g Carbohydrates: 24 g Fat: 4 g Sodium: 120 mg Potassium: 160 mg Phosphorus: 90 mg

### Procedure:

1. **Season Cucumber Slices:** In a small bowl, toss cucumber slices with lemon juice, black pepper, and a pinch of salt (if using).
2. **Assemble Sandwich:**
    - Toast the whole grain bread slices if desired.
    - Spread 1 tbsp of Dijon mustard on each slice of bread.
    - Place lettuce leaves on one bread slice.
    - Layer roasted turkey slices, seasoned cucumber slices, and shredded carrots over the lettuce.
    - Top with another bread slice.
3. **Serve:** Cut each sandwich in half and serve with a side salad or fruit.

### Batch Cooking and Meal Prepping Tips:

- **Pre-Slice Turkey:** Thinly slice extra roasted turkey breast ahead of time and store in the fridge for up to 3 days.
- **Prepare Vegetables:** Pre-slice cucumber and shred carrots in advance to make assembly quicker.
- **Wrap Individually:** Assemble sandwiches and wrap them individually for easy grab-and-go meals.

# Tuna Salad with Bell Peppers

- **Preparation Time:** 10 minutes
- **Servings:** 2

## Ingredients:

- 1 can (5 oz or 140 g) tuna packed in water, drained
- ½ medium red bell pepper, diced
- ½ medium yellow bell pepper, diced
- 2 tbsp (30 ml) plain Greek yogurt or low-fat mayonnaise
- 1 tsp (5 ml) Dijon mustard
- 1 tsp (5 ml) lemon juice
- ¼ tsp (1.25 ml) black pepper
- Pinch of salt (if allowed)
- 1 tbsp (15 g) scallions, finely chopped
- 1 tbsp (15 g) fresh parsley or cilantro, chopped
- 4 lettuce leaves for serving

## Nutritional Values (per serving):

Calories: 130 Protein: 15 g Carbohydrates: 8 g Fat: 3 g Sodium: 100 mg Potassium: 200 mg Phosphorus: 90 mg

## Procedure:

1. **Prep Ingredients:** Dice the bell peppers and chop the scallions and parsley or cilantro.
2. **Mix Dressing:** In a bowl, mix Greek yogurt or mayonnaise, Dijon mustard, lemon juice, black pepper, and salt (if using).
3. **Combine Salad:** Add the drained tuna, diced bell peppers, chopped scallions, and parsley or cilantro to the dressing. Mix until well combined. Adjust seasoning to taste.
4. **Serve:** Divide the tuna salad between two servings and enjoy with lettuce leaves as wraps or on whole grain bread.

## Batch Cooking and Meal Prepping Tips:

- **Prepare Tuna in Advance:** Drain and flake multiple cans of tuna and store them in an airtight container in the fridge.
- **Pre-Chop Vegetables:** Dice the bell peppers and chop the scallions and parsley or cilantro in advance to speed up salad assembly.
- **Make Extra Salad:** Double the recipe and store in individual portions for quick grab-and-go lunches.

# Black Bean Salsa with Pita

- **Preparation Time:** 10 minutes
- **Servings:** 2

## Ingredients:

- 1 can (15 oz or 425 g) black beans, drained and rinsed
- ½ cup (75 g) diced red bell pepper
- ½ cup (75 g) diced cucumber
- ¼ cup (35 g) diced red onion
- 1 medium tomato, diced
- 1 tbsp (15 ml) olive oil
- 2 tbsp (30 ml) lemon or lime juice
- 1 tsp (5 ml) cumin powder
- ½ tsp (2.5 ml) paprika
- ¼ tsp (1.25 ml) black pepper
- Pinch of salt (if allowed)
- 2 tbsp (30 g) chopped fresh cilantro or parsley
- 2 whole wheat pita breads

**Nutritional Values (per serving):**

Calories: 200 Protein: 8 g Carbohydrates: 30 g Fat: 4 g Sodium: 80 mg Potassium: 180 mg Phosphorus: 70 mg

## Procedure:

1. **Combine Vegetables:** In a large bowl, mix together the drained black beans, diced bell pepper, cucumber, red onion, and tomato.
2. **Prepare Dressing:** In a separate bowl, whisk together olive oil, lemon or lime juice, cumin, paprika, black pepper, and salt (if using).
3. **Mix Salsa:** Pour the dressing over the vegetable mixture and stir well to combine. Add the chopped cilantro or parsley and mix again. Adjust seasoning to taste.
4. **Serve with Pita:** Warm the pita breads in a skillet or toaster and cut them into triangles. Serve the salsa alongside the pita as a dip or filling.

## Batch Cooking and Meal Prepping Tips:

- **Pre-Chop Ingredients:** Dice the bell peppers, cucumber, red onion, and tomato ahead of time and store them in the fridge for up to 2 days.
- **Make Extra Salsa:** Double the recipe and store in airtight containers for up to 3 days.
- **Portion Pita:** Cut the pita into triangles and store them in resealable bags to keep them fresh for multiple servings.

# Couscous Salad with Mint and Lemon

- **Preparation Time:** 10 minutes
- **Cooking Time:** 5 minutes
- **Servings:** 4

### Ingredients:

- 1 cup (180 g) whole wheat couscous
- 1 cup (240 ml) water or low-sodium vegetable broth
- 2 tbsp (30 ml) olive oil
- 2 tbsp (30 ml) lemon juice
- 1 tsp (5 ml) lemon zest
- ½ tsp (2.5 ml) black pepper
- Pinch of salt (if allowed)
- ½ cup (75 g) diced cucumber
- ½ cup (75 g) diced bell pepper (any color)
- ¼ cup (35 g) diced red onion
- 2 tbsp (30 g) chopped fresh mint
- 2 tbsp (30 g) chopped fresh parsley

### Nutritional Values (per serving):

Calories: 180 Protein: 4 g Carbohydrates: 28 g Fat: 6 g Sodium: 40 mg Potassium: 160 mg Phosphorus: 60 mg

### Procedure:

1. **Cook Couscous:**
   - In a medium saucepan, bring the water or vegetable broth to a boil.
   - Stir in the couscous, cover, and remove from heat. Let it sit for 5 minutes, then fluff with a fork.
2. **Combine Vegetables:** In a large bowl, mix the diced cucumber, bell pepper, and red onion.
3. **Prepare Dressing:** In a separate bowl, whisk together olive oil, lemon juice, lemon zest, black pepper, and salt (if using).
4. **Mix Salad:** Add the cooked couscous to the bowl with the vegetables. Pour the dressing over the mixture and toss well to combine.
5. **Garnish & Serve:** Add the chopped mint and parsley and mix gently. Adjust seasoning to taste, and serve chilled or at room temperature.

### Batch Cooking and Meal Prepping Tips:

- **Make Extra Couscous:** Cook extra couscous to use in other salads or as a side dish for various meals.
- **Pre-Chop Vegetables:** Dice the cucumber, bell pepper, and onion in advance and store in airtight containers for quick assembly.

# Chicken Lettuce Wraps with Shredded Carrots

- **Preparation Time:** 10 minutes
- **Cooking Time:** 10 minutes
- **Servings:** 4

**Ingredients:**

- 1 lb (450 g) ground chicken
- 1 tbsp (15 ml) olive oil
- 2 garlic cloves, minced
- 1 tsp (5 ml) ginger, grated
- 1 tsp (5 ml) soy sauce or low-sodium tamari
- ¼ tsp (1.25 ml) black pepper
- Pinch of salt (if allowed)
- 1 cup (150 g) shredded carrots
- 1 cup (150 g) diced cucumber
- 1 tbsp (15 g) scallions, chopped
- 2 tbsp (30 g) fresh cilantro, chopped
- 8-10 leaves of butter or iceberg lettuce

**Nutritional Values (per serving):**

Calories: 180 Protein: 20 g Carbohydrates: 6 g Fat: 8 g Sodium: 120 mg Potassium: 180 mg Phosphorus: 80 mg

**Procedure:**

1. **Cook Chicken:** In a large skillet, heat olive oil over medium heat. Add the ground chicken and cook for 5-7 minutes, breaking it apart with a spatula until no longer pink.
2. **Add Aromatics:** Stir in the minced garlic and grated ginger. Cook for 1-2 minutes until fragrant.
3. **Season Chicken:** Add soy sauce or tamari, hoisin sauce (if using), black pepper, and salt (if allowed). Mix well and cook for another 2 minutes. Remove from heat.
4. **Assemble Wraps:** Place a generous spoonful of chicken mixture in each lettuce leaf. Top with shredded carrots, diced cucumber, chopped scallions, and fresh cilantro.
5. **Serve:** Arrange the wraps on a platter and serve immediately as appetizers or a light main course.

**Batch Cooking and Meal Prepping Tips:**

- **Prepare Chicken Mix:** Make a larger batch of ground chicken filling and store it in the fridge for up to 3 days.
- **Portion Control:** Pack chicken filling and lettuce leaves separately in meal prep containers for easy assembly during the week.

# Caprese Salad

- **Preparation Time:** 10 minutes
- **Servings:** 4

Ingredients:

- 4 medium ripe tomatoes, sliced
- 12 oz (340 g) fresh mozzarella, sliced
- 1 cup (15 g) fresh basil leaves
- 2 tbsp (30 ml) extra-virgin olive oil
- 1 tbsp (15 ml) balsamic glaze or balsamic vinegar
- ¼ tsp (1.25 ml) black pepper
- Pinch of salt (if allowed)

**Nutritional Values (per serving):**

Calories: 180 Protein: 9 g Carbohydrates: 6 g Fat: 14 g Sodium: 160 mg Potassium: 220 mg Phosphorus: 100 mg

**Procedure:**

1. **Slice Ingredients:** Slice the tomatoes and mozzarella into even-sized pieces.
2. **Layer Salad:** On a large serving platter, arrange alternating slices of tomato and mozzarella. Tuck fresh basil leaves between the slices.
3. **Drizzle Dressing:** Drizzle olive oil and balsamic glaze or vinegar over the salad.
4. **Season & Serve:** Sprinkle with black pepper and salt (if using) to taste. Serve immediately or chill for a few minutes before serving.

**Batch Cooking and Meal Prepping Tips:**

- **Pre-Slice Ingredients:** Slice the tomatoes and mozzarella in advance and store separately in airtight containers for up to 2 days.
- **Assemble Before Serving:** Assemble the salad just before serving to prevent it from becoming soggy.
- **Customize Flavor:** Add extra herbs like oregano or drizzle with pesto for a flavor twist.

# White Bean Stew with Low-Sodium Broth

- **Preparation Time:** 10 minutes
- **Cooking Time:** 30 minutes
- **Servings:** 4

### Ingredients:

- 1 tbsp (15 ml) olive oil
- 1 medium onion, diced
- 2 garlic cloves, minced
- 1 medium carrot, diced
- 1 celery stalk, diced
- 2 tsp (10 ml) ground cumin
- 1 tsp (5 ml) smoked paprika
- ½ tsp (2.5 ml) black pepper
- Pinch of salt (if allowed)
- 4 cups (1 L) low-sodium vegetable broth
- 2 cans (15 oz or 425 g each) white beans, drained and rinsed
- 1 can (14 oz or 400 g) diced tomatoes
- 2 bay leaves
- 2 tbsp (30 g) chopped fresh parsley or cilantro

### Nutritional Values (per serving):

Calories: 190 Protein: 10 g Carbohydrates: 30 g Fat: 5 g Sodium: 70 mg Potassium: 250 mg Phosphorus: 100 mg

### Procedure:

1. **Sauté Vegetables:** In a large pot, heat olive oil over medium heat. Add the diced onion, garlic, carrot, and celery. Sauté for 5-7 minutes until softened.
2. **Add Spices:** Add the cumin, smoked paprika, black pepper, and salt (if using). Stir well to coat the vegetables with the spices.
3. **Add Broth & Beans:** Add the low-sodium vegetable broth, white beans, diced tomatoes, and bay leaves. Stir to combine.
4. **Simmer Stew:** Bring to a gentle boil, then reduce the heat to low and let it simmer for 25-30 minutes until the flavors meld together.
5. **Finish & Serve:** Remove the bay leaves, stir in fresh parsley or cilantro, and adjust seasoning to taste. Ladle the stew into bowls and serve warm.

### Batch Cooking and Meal Prepping Tips:

- **Pre-Chop Vegetables:** Dice the onion, carrot, and celery ahead of time for quicker assembly.
- **Portion Control:** Divide the stew into individual containers for easy grab-and-go lunches or dinners.

# Orzo Pasta Salad with Tomatoes and Olives

- **Preparation Time:** 10 minutes
- **Cooking Time:** 10 minutes
- **Servings:** 4

### Ingredients:

- 1 cup (180 g) orzo pasta
- 1 tbsp (15 ml) olive oil
- 1 cup (150 g) cherry tomatoes, halved
- ½ cup (75 g) sliced black olives
- ¼ cup (35 g) diced cucumber
- ¼ cup (35 g) crumbled feta cheese (optional)
- 2 tbsp (30 g) fresh parsley or basil, chopped
- 2 tbsp (30 ml) lemon juice
- 1 tsp (5 ml) lemon zest
- ¼ tsp (1.25 ml) black pepper
- Pinch of salt (if allowed)

### Nutritional Values (per serving):

Calories: 150 Protein: 6 g Carbohydrates: 22 g Fat: 4 g Sodium: 100 mg Potassium: 130 mg Phosphorus: 60 mg

### Procedure:

1. **Cook Orzo:**
   - In a medium saucepan, bring salted water to a boil.
   - Add orzo pasta and cook according to package instructions (about 8-10 minutes) until al dente.
   - Drain and rinse under cold water to stop the cooking.

2. **Combine Vegetables:**
   - In a large bowl, mix together the halved cherry tomatoes, sliced black olives, diced cucumber, and crumbled feta cheese (if using).

3. **Prepare Dressing:**
   - In a separate bowl, whisk together olive oil, lemon juice, lemon zest, black pepper, and salt (if allowed).
   - **Assemble Salad:** Add the cooked orzo to the bowl with the vegetables. Pour the dressing over the mixture and toss well to combine.
   - **Garnish & Serve:** Add the chopped parsley or basil and mix gently. Adjust seasoning to taste and serve chilled or at room temperature.

# Zucchini Noodles with Turkey Meatballs

- **Preparation Time:** 15 minutes
- **Cooking Time:** 20 minutes
- **Servings:** 4

### Ingredients:

**Turkey Meatballs:**

- 1 lb (450 g) ground turkey
- 1 egg white
- 2 tbsp (30 g) breadcrumbs
- 1 garlic clove, minced
- 1 tbsp (15 g) fresh parsley, chopped
- ½ tsp (2.5 ml) paprika
- ¼ tsp (1.25 ml) black pepper
- Pinch of salt (if allowed)
- 1 tbsp (15 ml) olive oil

**Zucchini Noodles & Sauce:**

- 3-4 medium zucchini, spiralized into noodles
- 1 tbsp (15 ml) olive oil
- 2 garlic cloves, minced
- 1 can (14 oz or 400 g) diced tomatoes
- 1 tsp (5 ml) dried basil
- 2 tbsp (30 g) fresh basil, chopped

### Nutritional Values (per serving):

Calories: 180 Protein: 20 g Carbohydrates: 12 g Fat: 6 g Sodium: 110 mg Potassium: 180 mg Phosphorus: 80 mg

### Procedure:

**Make Meatballs: Prepare Mixture:** In a large bowl, mix ground turkey, egg white, breadcrumbs, minced garlic, parsley, paprika, black pepper, and salt (if using). Form the mixture into small, even-sized balls. **Cook Meatballs:** In a large skillet, heat olive oil over medium heat. Add the turkey meatballs and cook for 8-10 minutes, turning frequently, until browned and fully cooked. Transfer to a plate and set aside.

**Prepare Sauce & Noodles: Cook Sauce:** In the same skillet, add olive oil and minced garlic. Sauté for 1 minute until fragrant. Add the diced tomatoes, dried basil, black pepper, and salt (if using). Simmer for 10 minutes until slightly thickened. **Add Zucchini Noodles:** Add the spiralized zucchini noodles to the skillet with the sauce. Cook for 2-3 minutes until just tender.

**Assemble & Serve: Combine:** Add the cooked turkey meatballs back to the skillet and mix gently with the sauce and noodles. **Garnish:** Garnish with fresh basil before serving. Enjoy warm!

# Cauliflower Fried Rice with Peas

- **Preparation Time:** 10 minutes
- **Cooking Time:** 10 minutes
- **Servings:** 4

### Ingredients:

- 1 medium head of cauliflower, grated into "rice" (about 4 cups or 400 g)
- 1 tbsp (15 ml) olive oil
- 2 garlic cloves, minced
- 1 cup (150 g) frozen peas, thawed
- 2 large egg whites, lightly beaten
- 2 tbsp (30 ml) low-sodium soy sauce or tamari
- 1 tsp (5 ml) sesame oil (optional)
- ¼ tsp (1.25 ml) black pepper
- Pinch of salt (if allowed)
- 2 tbsp (30 g) scallions, chopped

### Nutritional Values (per serving):

Calories: 110 Protein: 6 g Carbohydrates: 15 g Fat: 4 g Sodium: 160 mg Potassium: 200 mg Phosphorus: 50 mg

### Procedure:

1. **Prepare Cauliflower:** Grate the cauliflower using a food processor or box grater until it resembles rice.
2. **Cook Garlic:** In a large skillet or wok, heat olive oil over medium-high heat. Add the minced garlic and sauté for 1-2 minutes until fragrant.
3. **Add Cauliflower:** Add the grated cauliflower to the skillet and stir-fry for 3-4 minutes until slightly softened.
4. **Add Peas & Egg Whites:** Add the peas and beaten egg whites to the skillet. Stir well to combine and cook for another 2-3 minutes until the eggs are set.
5. **Season & Garnish:** Add soy sauce or tamari, sesame oil (if using), black pepper, and salt (if allowed). Stir to mix and cook for another minute. Garnish with chopped scallions.
6. **Serve:** Divide the cauliflower fried rice between four bowls and serve warm.

### Batch Cooking and Meal Prepping Tips:

- **Make Ahead:** Cook a larger portion of the dish and store in meal prep containers in the fridge for up to 2 days.
- **Customize Flavor:** Add other low-potassium vegetables like bell peppers or carrots to diversify the flavors.

# Barley and Beet Salad

- **Preparation Time:** 15 minutes
- **Cooking Time:** 40 minutes
- **Servings:** 4

### Ingredients:

- 1 cup (180 g) pearl barley
- 2 cups (480 ml) water or low-sodium vegetable broth
- 3 medium beets, cooked and diced
- 1 medium cucumber, diced
- ¼ cup (35 g) crumbled feta cheese (optional)
- 2 tbsp (30 g) chopped fresh parsley or cilantro
- 2 tbsp (30 ml) lemon juice
- 2 tbsp (30 ml) olive oil
- 1 tsp (5 ml) Dijon mustard
- ½ tsp (2.5 ml) black pepper
- Pinch of salt (if allowed)

### Nutritional Values (per serving):

Calories: 180 Protein: 6 g Carbohydrates: 28 g Fat: 5 g Sodium: 80 mg Potassium: 160 mg Phosphorus: 80 mg

### Procedure:

1. **Cook Barley:**
   - In a medium saucepan, bring water or vegetable broth to a boil.
   - Add barley, reduce heat to low, and cover. Simmer for 30-40 minutes until tender.
   - Drain any excess liquid and let the barley cool.
2. **Prepare Beets:** If using raw beets, boil or steam them until tender. Once cooled, peel and dice them.
3. **Combine Vegetables:** In a large bowl, mix the cooked barley, diced beets, cucumber, and crumbled feta cheese (if using).
4. **Prepare Dressing:** In a small bowl, whisk together lemon juice, olive oil, Dijon mustard, black pepper, and salt (if allowed). **Mix Salad:** Pour the dressing over the barley mixture and toss well to combine.
5. **Garnish & Serve:** Add chopped parsley or cilantro and mix gently. Adjust seasoning to taste, and serve chilled or at room temperature.

### Batch Cooking and Meal Prepping Tips:

- **Pre-Cook Beets:** Cook and dice beets ahead of time and store them in the fridge to speed up assembly. **Portion Salad:** Divide the salad into individual containers for quick grab-and-go lunches or dinners.

# Sweet Potato and Spinach Quesadilla

- **Preparation Time:** 15 minutes
- **Cooking Time:** 20 minutes
- **Servings:** 4

## Ingredients:

- 2 medium sweet potatoes, peeled and diced
- 1 tbsp (15 ml) olive oil
- 2 cups (60 g) fresh spinach, roughly chopped
- 4 large whole wheat tortillas
- 1 cup (120 g) shredded cheese (such as mozzarella or cheddar)
- ½ tsp (2.5 ml) paprika
- ¼ tsp (1.25 ml) black pepper
- Pinch of salt (if allowed)

## Nutritional Values (per serving):

Calories: 180 Protein: 7 g Carbohydrates: 28 g Fat: 5 g Sodium: 90 mg Potassium: 150 mg Phosphorus: 80 mg

## Procedure:

1. **Cook Sweet Potatoes:**
   - In a medium saucepan, bring salted water to a boil.
   - Add the diced sweet potatoes and boil for 10-12 minutes until tender. Drain and mash them in a bowl.
   - Mix in paprika, black pepper, and salt (if using).

2. **Sauté Spinach:**
   - In a skillet, heat olive oil over medium heat.
   - Add the chopped spinach and sauté for 2-3 minutes until wilted.
   - Stir into the mashed sweet potatoes.

3. **Assemble Quesadilla:**
   - Place a tortilla on a flat surface and spread a layer of the sweet potato and spinach mixture evenly over one half.
   - Sprinkle with shredded cheese and fold the tortilla over to create a half-moon shape.
   - Repeat with remaining tortillas.
   - **Cook Quesadilla:** In a skillet over medium heat, lightly oil or spray with cooking spray. Add the quesadilla and cook for 2-3 minutes per side until golden brown and the cheese is melted.
   - **Serve:** Slice each quesadilla into wedges and serve immediately.

# Rice Noodle Salad with Shrimp

- **Preparation Time:** 15 minutes
- **Cooking Time:** 10 minutes
- **Servings:** 4

**Ingredients:**

- 8 oz (225 g) rice noodles
- 1 lb (450 g) shrimp, peeled and deveined
- 1 tbsp (15 ml) olive oil
- 1 tbsp (15 ml) lemon juice
- ½ tsp (2.5 ml) black pepper
- Pinch of salt (if allowed)
- 1 medium cucumber, sliced
- 1 cup (150 g) shredded carrots
- 1 cup (150 g) bean sprouts
- ¼ cup (35 g) chopped fresh cilantro
- 2 tbsp (30 ml) soy sauce or low-sodium tamari
- 2 tbsp (30 ml) rice vinegar
- 1 tsp (5 ml) sesame oil (optional)
- 1 tbsp (15 ml) lime juice

**Nutritional Values (per serving):**

Calories: 180 Protein: 18 g Carbohydrates: 20 g Fat: 4 g Sodium: 140 mg Potassium: 200 mg Phosphorus: 90 mg

**Procedure:**

1. **Cook Rice Noodles:**
   - In a large pot of boiling water, cook the rice noodles according to the package instructions (usually 5-7 minutes).
   - Drain and rinse under cold water to prevent sticking. Set aside.
2. **Cook Shrimp:**
   - In a skillet, heat olive oil over medium-high heat.
   - Add the shrimp, lemon juice, black pepper, and salt (if allowed).
   - Sauté for 3-4 minutes until the shrimp is pink and opaque. Remove from heat and let it cool slightly.
   - **Prepare Salad:** In a large bowl, combine the rice noodles, cucumber slices, shredded carrots, bean sprouts, and cilantro. Add the cooked shrimp and mix well.
   - **Mix Dressing:** In a small bowl, whisk together soy sauce or tamari, rice vinegar, sesame oil (if using), and lime juice. Pour the dressing over the salad and toss well to combine.
   - **Serve:** Divide the salad among four bowls and serve immediately.

# Greek-Style Tabbouleh with Parsley and Lemon

- **Preparation Time:** 15 minutes
- **Cooking Time:** 10 minutes
- **Servings:** 4

## Ingredients:

- 1 cup (180 g) bulgur wheat
- 2 cups (480 ml) water or low-sodium vegetable broth
- 1 cup (150 g) cherry tomatoes, diced
- 1 cucumber, diced
- ½ cup (75 g) crumbled feta cheese (optional)
- 2 tbsp (30 g) chopped fresh mint
- 1 cup (30 g) chopped fresh parsley
- 3 tbsp (45 ml) lemon juice
- 3 tbsp (45 ml) olive oil
- 1 tsp (5 ml) lemon zest
- ½ tsp (2.5 ml) black pepper
- Pinch of salt (if allowed)

## Nutritional Values (per serving):

Calories: 190 Protein: 5 g Carbohydrates: 25 g Fat: 7 g Sodium: 90 mg Potassium: 130 mg Phosphorus: 60 mg

## Procedure:

1. **Cook Bulgur Wheat:**
    - In a medium saucepan, bring water or vegetable broth to a boil.
    - Add the bulgur wheat, cover, and reduce the heat to low. Simmer for 10 minutes until tender.
    - Drain any excess liquid, fluff with a fork, and let cool.
2. **Combine Vegetables:** In a large bowl, mix the diced cherry tomatoes, cucumber, crumbled feta cheese (if using), mint, and parsley.
    - **Prepare Dressing:** In a separate bowl, whisk together lemon juice, olive oil, lemon zest, black pepper, and salt (if using).
3. **Mix Tabbouleh:**
    - Add the cooled bulgur wheat to the bowl with the vegetables.
    - Pour the dressing over the mixture and toss well to combine.
    - **Garnish & Serve:** Adjust seasoning to taste, and serve the tabbouleh chilled or at room temperature.

# Dinner

## Baked Cod with Lemon and Dill Over Wild Rice

- **Preparation Time:** 10 minutes
- **Cooking Time:** 20 minutes
- **Servings:** 4

### Ingredients:

- 4 cod fillets (about 6 oz or 170 g each)
- 2 tbsp (30 ml) olive oil
- 2 tbsp (30 ml) lemon juice
- 2 tbsp (30 g) chopped fresh dill
- 1 tsp (5 ml) lemon zest
- ½ tsp (2.5 ml) black pepper
- Pinch of salt (if allowed)
- 1½ cups (270 g) wild rice
- 3 cups (720 ml) low-sodium vegetable broth or water

### Nutritional Values (per serving):

Calories: 220 Protein: 25 g Carbohydrates: 30 g Fat: 5 g Sodium: 80 mg Potassium: 160 mg Phosphorus: 100 mg

### Procedure:

**Cook Rice:**

- **Prepare Wild Rice:** In a medium saucepan, bring vegetable broth or water to a boil. Add the wild rice, cover, and reduce the heat to low. Simmer for 30-40 minutes until tender. Drain any excess liquid.

**Bake Cod:**

1. **Preheat Oven:** Preheat the oven to 400°F (200°C).
2. **Season Cod Fillets:**
   - In a small bowl, mix olive oil, lemon juice, lemon zest, black pepper, and salt (if allowed).
   - Brush the mixture over the cod fillets.
   - Place the fillets in a baking dish and sprinkle with chopped dill.
3. **Bake:** Bake the cod fillets for 12-15 minutes, or until the fish flakes easily with a fork.
4. **Assemble:**
   - Divide the cooked wild rice between four plates.
   - Place a baked cod fillet on top of each portion of rice.
   - Garnish with extra dill or lemon zest if desired, and serve warm.

# Grilled Salmon with Steamed Low-Potassium Vegetables and Quinoa

- **Preparation Time:** 15 minutes
- **Cooking Time:** 20 minutes
- **Servings:** 4

### Ingredients:

### Salmon and Vegetables:

- 4 salmon fillets (about 6 oz or 170 g each)
- 2 tbsp (30 ml) olive oil
- 1 tbsp (15 ml) lemon juice
- 1 tsp (5 ml) lemon zest
- ½ tsp (2.5 ml) black pepper
- Pinch of salt (if allowed)
- 2 cups (300 g) zucchini, sliced into rounds
- 1½ cups (225 g) bell peppers, cut into strips
- 1 cup (150 g) green beans

### Quinoa:

- 1 cup (170 g) quinoa, rinsed
- 2 cups (480 ml) water or low-sodium vegetable broth

### Nutritional Values (per serving):

Calories: 280 Protein: 30 g Carbohydrates: 24 g Fat: 8 g Sodium: 100 mg Potassium: 250 mg Phosphorus: 120 mg

### Procedure:

**Cook Quinoa:** In a medium saucepan, bring water or vegetable broth to a boil. Add the quinoa, reduce the heat to low, and cover. Simmer for 15 minutes until the quinoa is tender and has absorbed the liquid. Remove from heat and let it sit for 5 minutes, then fluff with a fork.

### Grill Salmon & Steam Vegetables:

1. **Preheat Grill:** Preheat your grill to medium-high heat.
    - **Season Salmon Fillets:** In a small bowl, mix olive oil, lemon juice, lemon zest, black pepper, and salt (if allowed).
    - Brush the mixture evenly over the salmon fillets.
    - **Grill Salmon:** Place the salmon fillets on the grill and cook for 3-4 minutes per side until the fish flakes easily with a fork.
2. **Steam Vegetables:** While the salmon is grilling, steam the zucchini, bell peppers, and green beans for 5-7 minutes until tender.

**Serve:** Divide the quinoa among four plates. Top with grilled salmon fillets and steamed vegetables. Serve immediately, garnished with extra lemon zest if desired.

# Herb-Crusted Chicken Breast with Sautéed Zucchini

- **Preparation Time:** 15 minutes
- **Cooking Time:** 20 minutes
- **Servings:** 4

## Ingredients:

### Herb-Crusted Chicken:

- 4 chicken breasts (about 6 oz or 170 g each)
- 2 tbsp (30 ml) olive oil
- 1 tsp (5 ml) lemon juice
- 1 tsp (5 ml) lemon zest
- 1 tbsp (15 ml) chopped fresh parsley
- 1 tbsp (15 ml) chopped fresh thyme
- 1 tsp (5 ml) black pepper

### Sautéed Zucchini:

- 2 tbsp (30 ml) olive oil
- 2 garlic cloves, minced
- 3 medium zucchini, sliced into rounds
- 1 tsp (5 ml) dried oregano
- 1 tsp (5 ml) black pepper
- Pinch of salt (if allowed)

## Nutritional Values (per serving):

Calories: 220 Protein: 28 g Carbohydrates: 10 g Fat: 8 g Sodium: 100 mg Potassium: 200 mg Phosphorus: 90 mg

## Procedure:

### Prepare Chicken:

1. **Preheat Oven:** Preheat the oven to 375°F (190°C).
2. **Mix Herb Coating:** In a small bowl, combine olive oil, Dijon mustard, lemon juice, lemon zest, parsley, thyme, black pepper, and salt (if using). Mix well.
3. **Coat Chicken:** Brush the herb mixture evenly over each chicken breast. Place the chicken breasts on a baking sheet lined with parchment paper. **Bake Chicken:** Bake for 15-20 minutes or until the chicken is fully cooked and reaches an internal temperature of 165°F (74°C).

### Sauté Zucchini:

- **Cook Zucchini:** In a large skillet, heat olive oil over medium-high heat. Add the minced garlic and sauté for 1 minute until fragrant. Add the zucchini slices, oregano, black pepper, and salt. Sauté for 5-7 minutes, stirring occasionally, until the zucchini is tender and lightly browned.

**Serve:** Divide the zucchini among four plates. Top each with a herb-crusted chicken breast.

# Stuffed Bell Peppers with Ground Turkey and Brown Rice

- **Preparation Time:** 15 minutes
- **Cooking Time:** 30 minutes
- **Servings:** 4

### Ingredients:

- 4 large bell peppers (any color), tops cut off and seeds removed
- 1 lb (450 g) ground turkey
- 1 cup (170 g) cooked brown rice
- 1 medium onion, diced
- 2 garlic cloves, minced
- 1 tbsp (15 ml) olive oil
- 1 tsp (5 ml) ground cumin
- ½ tsp (2.5 ml) paprika
- ½ tsp (2.5 ml) black pepper
- Pinch of salt (if allowed)
- 1 cup (150 g) diced tomatoes
- ¼ cup (60 g) shredded cheese (optional)
- 2 tbsp (30 g) chopped fresh parsley or cilantro

### Nutritional Values (per serving):

Calories: 230 Protein: 20 g Carbohydrates: 25 g Fat: 7 g Sodium: 80 mg Potassium: 180 mg Phosphorus: 90 mg

### Procedure:

**Prepare Bell Peppers:**

1. **Preheat Oven:** Preheat the oven to 375°F (190°C).
2. **Prep Peppers:** Cut the tops off the bell peppers and remove the seeds. Lightly oil the outside of the peppers and place them in a baking dish.

**Cook Filling:**

- **Sauté Vegetables:** In a skillet, heat olive oil over medium heat. Add the diced onion and garlic. Sauté for 3-4 minutes until softened.
- **Add Turkey & Spices:** Add the ground turkey, cumin, paprika, black pepper, and salt (if using). Cook for 5-7 minutes, breaking up the turkey, until fully cooked.
- **Mix Filling:** Add the cooked brown rice and diced tomatoes to the skillet. Stir well to combine.
- **Stuff Peppers:** Spoon the filling into the prepared bell peppers. If desired, sprinkle shredded cheese on top of each pepper.
- **Bake Peppers:** Cover the baking dish with aluminum foil and bake for 25-30 minutes until the peppers are tender. Remove the foil during the last 5 minutes of baking for a crispier cheese topping. **Serve:** Serve warm and enjoy!

# Braised Tofu with Bok Choy and Sesame Oil

- **Preparation Time:** 15 minutes
- **Cooking Time:** 20 minutes
- **Servings:** 4

### Ingredients:

- 1 lb (450 g) firm tofu, drained and cut into cubes
- 1 tbsp (15 ml) sesame oil
- 2 tbsp (30 ml) soy sauce or tamari (low-sodium if available)
- 1 tbsp (15 ml) rice vinegar
- 2 tsp (10 ml) honey or maple syrup
- 2 garlic cloves, minced
- 1 tbsp (15 ml) grated ginger
- 1 tbsp (15 ml) vegetable oil
- 1 medium onion, sliced
- 4 cups (300 g) bok choy, chopped
- ½ tsp (2.5 ml) black pepper
- 1 tbsp (15 g) sesame seeds
- 2 tbsp (30 g) chopped scallions

### Nutritional Values (per serving):

Calories: 170 Protein: 12 g Carbohydrates: 10 g Fat: 8 g Sodium: 130 mg Potassium: 200 mg Phosphorus: 60 mg

### Procedure:

**Prepare Tofu Marinade:**

- **Make Marinade:** In a small bowl, whisk together sesame oil, soy sauce or tamari, rice vinegar, honey or maple syrup, minced garlic, and grated ginger.
- **Marinate Tofu:** Add the tofu cubes to the marinade and let them sit for 10 minutes.

**Cook Tofu & Vegetables:**

- **Sear Tofu:** In a large skillet, heat vegetable oil over medium-high heat. Add the marinated tofu and sear for 3-4 minutes per side until golden brown. Remove and set aside.
- **Sauté Onion:** In the same skillet, add the sliced onion and cook for 5 minutes until softened.
- **Add Bok Choy:** Add the chopped bok choy, black pepper, and a splash of water or broth. Stir well and cook for 3-4 minutes until the bok choy is tender but still crisp.
- **Combine & Braise:** Return the tofu to the skillet and pour in the remaining marinade. Cook for another 5 minutes, stirring occasionally, to allow the flavors to blend. Serve warm.

# Shrimp Stir-Fry with Snow Peas and Jasmine Rice

- **Preparation Time:** 15 minutes
- **Cooking Time:** 15 minutes
- **Servings:** 4

## Ingredients:

### Stir-Fry:

- 1 lb (450 g) shrimp, peeled and deveined
- 1 tbsp (15 ml) soy sauce or tamari (low-sodium)
- 2 tbsp (30 ml) vegetable oil
- 2 garlic cloves, minced
- 1 tbsp (15 ml) grated ginger
- 1½ cups (270 g) jasmine rice
- 1 cup (150 g) snow peas, trimmed
- 1 red bell pepper, julienned
- 1 tsp (5 ml) sesame oil
- ¼ tsp (1.25 ml) black pepper
- Pinch of salt (if allowed)
- 3 cups (720 ml) water or low-sodium vegetable broth

## Nutritional Values (per serving):

Calories: 240 Protein: 18 g Carbohydrates: 32 g Fat: 6 g Sodium: 140 mg Potassium: 200 mg Phosphorus: 90 mg

## Procedure:

### Prepare Jasmine Rice:

- **Cook Rice:** In a medium saucepan, bring water or vegetable broth to a boil. Add the jasmine rice, reduce heat to low, and cover. Simmer for 15 minutes until tender and the liquid is absorbed. Fluff the rice with a fork and keep it covered until ready to serve.

### Cook Shrimp Stir-Fry:

- **Season Shrimp:** Toss the peeled shrimp with soy sauce or tamari.
- **Stir-Fry Shrimp:** In a large skillet or wok, heat vegetable oil over medium-high heat. Add the shrimp and stir-fry for 2-3 minutes until pink and opaque. Remove the shrimp from the skillet and set aside.
- **Cook Vegetables:** Add the minced garlic and grated ginger to the skillet. Sauté for 1 minute until fragrant, then add the snow peas and bell pepper. Stir-fry for 4-5 minutes until the vegetables are tender but still crisp.
- **Combine & Season:** Return the shrimp to the skillet and stir in sesame oil, black pepper, and salt (if allowed). Top with the shrimp stir-fry and serve immediately.

# Chicken and Vegetable Kebabs with Couscous

- **Preparation Time:** 15 minutes
- **Cooking Time:** 20 minutes
- **Servings:** 4

**Ingredients:**

**Kebabs:**

- 1 lb (450 g) boneless, skinless chicken breast, cut into cubes
- 1 red bell pepper, cut into chunks
- 1 medium zucchini, cut into thick slices
- 1 medium red onion, cut into chunks
- 1 tbsp (15 ml) olive oil
- 1 tsp (5 ml) paprika
- 1 tsp (5 ml) ground cumin
- ½ tsp (2.5 ml) black pepper
- Pinch of salt (if allowed)
- 2 tbsp (30 ml) lemon juice
- Wooden skewers, soaked in water

**Couscous:**

- 1 cup (180 g) couscous
- 1½ cups (360 ml) water or low-sodium vegetable broth
- 1 tbsp (15 ml) olive oil
- 1 tbsp (15 ml) lemon juice
- 1 tsp (5 ml) lemon zest
- ¼ tsp (1.25 ml) black pepper
- Pinch of salt (if allowed)
- 2 tbsp (30 g) chopped parsley

**Nutritional Values (per serving):**

Calories: 230 Protein: 25 g Carbohydrates: 26 g Fat: 6 g Sodium: 120 mg Potassium: 200 mg Phosphorus: 110 mg

**Procedure:**

**Prepare Kebabs: Preheat Grill:** Preheat your grill to medium-high heat.

- **Season Chicken & Vegetables:** In a large bowl, combine olive oil, paprika, cumin, black pepper, salt (if using), and lemon juice. Add the cubed chicken, bell peppers, zucchini, and onion to the bowl and toss to coat evenly. **Assemble Kebabs:** Thread the marinated chicken and vegetables onto the wooden skewers, alternating them.
- **Grill Kebabs:** Place the skewers on the grill and cook for 10-12 minutes, turning occasionally, until the chicken is fully cooked and the vegetables are lightly charred.

**Cook Couscous:** In a medium saucepan, bring water or vegetable broth to a boil. Add the couscous, cover, and remove from heat. Let it sit for 5 minutes. Serve warm.

# Mushroom Risotto with Herbs

- **Preparation Time:** 15 minutes
- **Cooking Time:** 30 minutes
- **Servings:** 4

**Ingredients:**

- 1½ cups (280 g) Arborio rice
- 6 cups (1.4 L) low-sodium vegetable broth
- 2 tbsp (30 ml) olive oil
- 1 medium onion, diced
- 2 garlic cloves, minced
- 2 cups (300 g) mushrooms, sliced
- ½ cup (120 ml) dry white wine (optional)
- 1 tsp (5 ml) black pepper
- Pinch of salt (if allowed)
- ½ cup (60 g) grated Parmesan cheese (optional)
- 2 tbsp (30 g) chopped fresh parsley
- 1 tbsp (15 g) chopped fresh thyme

**Nutritional Values (per serving):**

Calories: 250 Protein: 8 g Carbohydrates: 40 g Fat: 8 g Sodium: 120 mg Potassium: 150 mg Phosphorus: 100 mg

**Procedure:**

1. **Warm Broth:** In a medium saucepan, warm the vegetable broth over low heat and keep it at a gentle simmer.
2. **Sauté Onion & Garlic:** In a large skillet, heat the olive oil over medium heat. Add the diced onion and sauté for 5 minutes until softened. Add the minced garlic and cook for another minute until fragrant.
3. **Cook Mushrooms:** Add the sliced mushrooms to the skillet and cook for 5-7 minutes until softened.
4. **Add Rice & Wine:** Add the Arborio rice to the skillet and stir to coat it with oil. Cook for 2 minutes until the rice becomes slightly translucent. Pour in the white wine (if using) and cook, stirring constantly, until it evaporates.
5. **Add Broth:** Ladle in the warm vegetable broth, one cup at a time, stirring frequently. Wait for each cup of broth to be absorbed before adding the next. Continue this process until the rice is creamy and tender, about 20 minutes.
6. **Finish & Serve:** Stir in the black pepper, salt (if using), grated Parmesan (if using), parsley, and thyme. Adjust seasoning to taste and serve warm.

# Baked Tilapia with Lemon and Garlic Green Beans

- **Preparation Time:** 15 minutes
- **Cooking Time:** 20 minutes
- **Servings:** 4

**Ingredients:**

**Baked Tilapia:**

- 4 tilapia fillets (about 6 oz or 170 g each)
- 2 tbsp (30 ml) olive oil
- 1 tbsp (15 ml) lemon juice
- 1 tsp (5 ml) lemon zest
- 1 tsp (5 ml) paprika
- ½ tsp (2.5 ml) black pepper
- Pinch of salt (if allowed)

**Garlic Green Beans:**

- 2 tbsp (30 ml) olive oil
- 2 garlic cloves, minced
- 1 lb (450 g) green beans, trimmed
- 1 tsp (5 ml) lemon juice
- ½ tsp (2.5 ml) black pepper
- Pinch of salt (if allowed)

**Nutritional Values (per serving):** Calories: 220 Protein: 30 g Carbohydrates: 10 g Fat: 8 g Sodium: 120 mg Potassium: 170 mg Phosphorus: 100 mg

**Procedure:**

**Bake Tilapia: Preheat Oven:** Preheat the oven to 400°F (200°C).

1. **Season Tilapia:** In a small bowl, mix olive oil, lemon juice, lemon zest, paprika, black pepper, and salt (if using). Brush the mixture evenly over the tilapia fillets.
2. **Bake Fillets:** Place the seasoned fillets on a baking sheet lined with parchment paper. Bake for 12-15 minutes or until the fish flakes easily with a fork.

**Prepare Green Beans:**

1. **Sauté Garlic:** In a large skillet, heat olive oil over medium heat. Add the minced garlic and sauté for 1-2 minutes until fragrant.
2. **Cook Green Beans:** Add the trimmed green beans to the skillet and stir to coat them with the garlic-infused oil. Cook for 5-7 minutes, stirring occasionally, until the beans are tender but still crisp.
3. **Season Beans:** Stir in lemon juice, black pepper, and salt (if using). Cook for another 1-2 minutes, then remove from heat. **Serve:** Divide the baked tilapia and garlic green beans among four plates. Serve warm and enjoy immediately.

# Turkey Chili with Kidney Beans

- **Preparation Time:** 15 minutes
- **Cooking Time:** 30 minutes
- **Servings:** 4

**Ingredients:**

- 1 lb (450 g) ground turkey
- 1 tbsp (15 ml) olive oil
- 1 medium onion, diced
- 2 garlic cloves, minced
- 1 red bell pepper, diced
- 2 tsp (10 ml) ground cumin
- 2 tsp (10 ml) chili powder
- 1 tsp (5 ml) smoked paprika
- ½ tsp (2.5 ml) black pepper
- Pinch of salt (if allowed)
- 2 cups (480 ml) low-sodium vegetable broth
- 1 can (15 oz or 425 g) diced tomatoes
- 1 can (15 oz or 425 g) kidney beans, drained and rinsed
- 1 tbsp (15 ml) tomato paste
- 1 tsp (5 ml) hot sauce (optional)
- 2 tbsp (30 g) chopped fresh cilantro

**Nutritional Values (per serving):**

Calories: 220 Protein: 20 g Carbohydrates: 22 g Fat: 7 g Sodium: 80 mg Potassium: 210 mg Phosphorus: 90 mg

**Procedure:**

1. **Cook Turkey:** In a large pot or Dutch oven, heat olive oil over medium heat. Add the ground turkey and cook for 5-7 minutes, breaking it apart with a spatula, until no longer pink.
2. **Sauté Vegetables:** Add the diced onion, minced garlic, and diced bell pepper. Sauté for 5 minutes until the vegetables are softened.
3. **Add Spices:** Add ground cumin, chili powder, smoked paprika, black pepper, and salt (if using). Stir well to coat the vegetables and turkey with the spices.
4. **Add Liquids & Beans:** Pour in vegetable broth, diced tomatoes, kidney beans, tomato paste, and hot sauce (if using). Stir to combine, then bring to a boil. Reduce heat to low and let it simmer for 20 minutes, stirring occasionally.
5. **Finish & Serve:** Stir in chopped cilantro before serving. Adjust seasoning to taste, and serve warm with your favorite toppings like avocado or shredded cheese.

# Lentil Loaf with Mashed Sweet Potatoes

**Preparation Time:** 20 minutes  •  **Cooking Time:** 45 minutes  •  **Servings:** 4

**Ingredients:**

**Lentil Loaf:**

- 1 cup (200 g) dried green or brown lentils, rinsed and drained
- 2 cups (480 ml) water or low-sodium vegetable broth
- 1 tbsp (15 ml) olive oil
- 1 medium onion, diced
- 2 garlic cloves, minced
- 1 medium carrot, diced
- 1 celery stalk, diced
- 1 tsp (5 ml) ground cumin
- 1 tsp (5 ml) smoked paprika
- ½ tsp (2.5 ml) black pepper
- Pinch of salt (if allowed)
- ½ cup (50 g) breadcrumbs
- ¼ cup (30 g) ground flaxseed
- 2 tbsp (30 ml) tomato paste
- 2 tbsp (30 g) chopped fresh parsley

**Mashed Sweet Potatoes:**

- 2 large sweet potatoes, peeled and diced
- 2 tbsp (30 ml) olive oil or unsalted butter
- 1 tsp (5 ml) ground cinnamon
- ¼ tsp (1.25 ml) black pepper
- Pinch of salt (if allowed)

**Procedure:**

**Prepare Lentil Loaf: Cook Lentils:** In a medium saucepan, bring water or vegetable broth to a boil. Add the lentils, reduce heat, cover, and simmer for 20-25 minutes until tender. Drain and set aside.

**Sauté Vegetables:** In a skillet, heat olive oil over medium heat. Add diced onion, garlic, carrot, and celery. Sauté for 5-7 minutes until softened.

**Combine Loaf Mixture:** In a large bowl, combine cooked lentils, sautéed vegetables, cumin, paprika, black pepper, and salt (if using). Add breadcrumbs, ground flaxseed, tomato paste, and parsley. Mix well until the mixture holds together.

**Bake Loaf:** Preheat the oven to 375°F (190°C). Press the mixture into a greased loaf pan. Bake for 30-35 minutes until firm.

**Prepare Mashed Sweet Potatoes: Boil Sweet Potatoes:** In a large pot, bring salted water to a boil. Add diced sweet potatoes and boil for 12-15 minutes until tender. Drain well.
**Mash and Serve.**

# Grilled Lamb Chops with Roasted Brussels Sprouts

- **Preparation Time:** 15 minutes
- **Cooking Time:** 25 minutes
- **Servings:** 4

**Ingredients:**

**Grilled Lamb Chops:**

- 8 lamb chops (about 3 oz or 85 g each)
- 2 tbsp (30 ml) olive oil
- 1 tbsp (15 ml) lemon juice
- 2 garlic cloves, minced
- 1 tbsp (15 ml) chopped fresh rosemary
- 1 tsp (5 ml) black pepper

**Roasted Brussels Sprouts:**

- 1 lb (450 g) Brussels sprouts, trimmed and halved
- 2 tbsp (30 ml) olive oil
- 1 tsp (5 ml) balsamic vinegar
- 1 tsp (5 ml) black pepper
- Pinch of salt (if allowed)

**Nutritional Values (per serving):**

Calories: 250 Protein: 25 g Carbohydrates: 10 g Fat: 12 g Sodium: 90 mg Potassium: 180 mg Phosphorus: 100 mg

**Procedure:**

**Prepare Brussels Sprouts:**

1. **Preheat Oven:** Preheat the oven to 400°F (200°C).
2. **Season Brussels Sprouts:**
   - In a bowl, toss Brussels sprouts with olive oil, balsamic vinegar, black pepper, and salt (if allowed).
   - Spread them evenly on a baking sheet.

**Roast:** Roast for 20-25 minutes, stirring halfway through, until the sprouts are golden and slightly crispy.

**Prepare Lamb Chops:**

- **Marinate Lamb Chops:** In a small bowl, mix olive oil, lemon juice, garlic, rosemary, black pepper, and salt (if using). Rub the mixture over the lamb chops and let them sit for at least 10 minutes.
- **Grill Lamb Chops:** Preheat the grill to medium-high heat. Grill the lamb chops for 2-3 minutes per side, depending on thickness, until they reach your desired level of doneness. Place two grilled lamb chops on each plate, and serve immediately.

# Vegetable Paella with Parsley

- **Preparation Time:** 15 minutes
- **Cooking Time:** 30 minutes
- **Servings:** 4

### Ingredients:

- 2 tbsp (30 ml) olive oil
- 1 medium onion, diced
- 2 garlic cloves, minced
- 1 medium red bell pepper, diced
- 1 medium zucchini, diced
- 1½ cups (280 g) Arborio or short-grain rice
- 2 tsp (10 ml) smoked paprika
- 1 tsp (5 ml) ground cumin
- ½ tsp (2.5 ml) saffron threads (optional)
- ½ tsp (2.5 ml) black pepper
- Pinch of salt (if allowed)
- 4 cups (1 L) low-sodium vegetable broth
- 1 cup (150 g) green peas, frozen or fresh
- 2 tbsp (30 g) chopped fresh parsley
- Lemon wedges for garnish

### Nutritional Values (per serving):

Calories: 220 Protein: 7 g Carbohydrates: 38 g Fat: 5 g Sodium: 80 mg Potassium: 150 mg Phosphorus: 70 mg

### Procedure:

1. **Sauté Vegetables:**
   - In a large skillet or paella pan, heat olive oil over medium heat.
   - Add the diced onion and minced garlic and sauté for 5 minutes until softened.
   - Add the diced red bell pepper and zucchini, and cook for another 3-4 minutes.

2. **Add Spices & Rice:**
   - Stir in smoked paprika, ground cumin, saffron threads (if using), black pepper, and salt (if allowed).
   - Add the Arborio rice and stir to coat it with the spices.
   - **Add Broth:** Pour in the vegetable broth and bring it to a boil. Reduce heat to low and simmer for 20 minutes, stirring occasionally, until the rice is tender and has absorbed most of the liquid.

3. **Add Peas & Parsley and Serve warm.**

# Spinach and Ricotta-Stuffed Chicken Breast

- **Preparation Time:** 20 minutes
- **Cooking Time:** 30 minutes
- **Servings:** 4

## Ingredients:

- 4 boneless, skinless chicken breasts (about 6 oz or 170 g each)
- 2 tbsp (30 ml) olive oil
- 1 tsp (5 ml) black pepper
- Pinch of salt (if allowed)

## Stuffing:

- 2 cups (60 g) fresh spinach, chopped
- ½ cup (120 g) ricotta cheese
- ¼ cup (30 g) grated Parmesan cheese (optional)
- 2 garlic cloves, minced
- 1 tsp (5 ml) dried oregano
- ½ tsp (2.5 ml) black pepper

## Nutritional Values (per serving):

Calories: 220 Protein: 30 g Carbohydrates: 5 g Fat: 8 g Sodium: 120 mg Potassium: 180 mg Phosphorus: 90 mg

## Procedure:

**Mix Ingredients:** In a medium bowl, mix the chopped spinach, ricotta cheese, Parmesan cheese (if using), minced garlic, dried oregano, and black pepper until well combined.

## Prepare Chicken:

1. **Preheat Oven:** Preheat the oven to 375°F (190°C).
2. **Slice Chicken Breasts:** Using a sharp knife, cut a pocket into each chicken breast, being careful not to slice through.
3. **Stuff Chicken Breasts:** Fill each pocket with a generous amount of the spinach and ricotta mixture. Secure the opening with toothpicks if needed.
4. **Season Chicken:** Brush the chicken breasts with olive oil and season with black pepper and salt (if allowed).

## Bake Chicken:

1. **Bake in Oven:** Place the stuffed chicken breasts in a baking dish and cover with foil. Bake for 20-25 minutes until the chicken is fully cooked and reaches an internal temperature of 165°F (74°C).

**Remove Foil:** Remove the foil and bake for an additional 5 minutes to lightly brown the top. Serve warm with your favorite side dish.

# Quinoa-Stuffed Acorn Squash

- **Preparation Time:** 20 minute
- **Cooking Time:** 40 minutes
- **Servings:** 4

**Ingredients:**

**Acorn Squash:**

- 2 acorn squash, halved and seeds removed
- 2 tbsp (30 ml) olive oil
- 1 tsp (5 ml) black pepper
- Pinch of salt (if allowed)

**Quinoa Filling:**

- 1 cup (170 g) quinoa, rinsed
- 2 cups (480 ml) low-sodium vegetable broth or water
- 2 tbsp (30 ml) olive oil
- 1 medium onion, diced
- 1 garlic clove, minced
- 1 cup (150 g) diced mushrooms
- ½ cup (75 g) diced bell pepper
- ½ cup (75 g) dried cranberries
- 1 tsp (5 ml) ground cumin
- ½ tsp (2.5 ml) smoked paprika
- 1 tsp (5 ml) black pepper
- Pinch of salt (if allowed)
- ¼ cup (35 g) chopped fresh parsley

**Procedure:**

**Prepare Squash:**

1. **Preheat Oven:** Preheat the oven to 400°F (200°C).
2. **Season & Roast:** Brush the inside of the acorn squash halves with olive oil and season with black pepper and salt (if allowed). Place the halves cut-side down on a baking sheet and roast for 30-35 minutes until tender.

**Prepare Quinoa Filling:**

1. **Cook Quinoa:** In a medium saucepan, bring the vegetable broth or water to a boil. Add the rinsed quinoa, cover, and reduce heat to low. Simmer for 15 minutes until the quinoa is tender and has absorbed the liquid. Fluff with a fork and set aside.
2. **Sauté Vegetables:** In a skillet, heat olive oil over medium heat. Add diced onion and minced garlic, and sauté for 5 minutes until softened. Add the mushrooms and bell pepper, and cook for another 5 minutes.

**Mix Filling:** Add the cooked quinoa, dried cranberries, cumin, paprika, black pepper, and salt (if allowed) to the skillet. Stir well to combine and cook for 2-3 minutes.
**Assemble & Serve**

# Broiled Flank Steak with Barley

- **Preparation Time:** 15 minutes
- **Cooking Time:** 40 minutes
- **Servings:** 4

**Ingredients:**

**Flank Steak:**

- 1 lb (450 g) flank steak
- 2 tbsp (30 ml) olive oil
- 1 tbsp (15 ml) soy sauce or tamari (low-sodium if available)
- 1 tbsp (15 ml) lemon juice
- 1 tsp (5 ml) paprika
- 1 tsp (5 ml) black pepper
- Pinch of salt (if allowed)

**Barley:**

- 1 cup (180 g) pearl barley
- 3 cups (720 ml) low-sodium vegetable broth or water
- 1 tbsp (15 ml) olive oil
- 1 tsp (5 ml) lemon zest
- 1 tsp (5 ml) black pepper
- Pinch of salt (if allowed)
- 2 tbsp (30 g) chopped fresh parsley

**Nutritional Values (per serving):** Calories: 250 Protein: 22 g Carbohydrates: 28 g Fat: 8 g Sodium: 110 mg Potassium: 170 mg Phosphorus: 90 mg

**Procedure:**

**Prepare Flank Steak:**

1. **Marinate Steak:** In a small bowl, combine olive oil, soy sauce or tamari, lemon juice, paprika, black pepper, and salt (if allowed). Rub the mixture over the flank steak and let it sit for at least 15 minutes.
2. **Preheat Broiler:** Preheat your broiler to high heat.
3. **Broil Steak:** Place the marinated flank steak on a broiler pan or baking sheet. Broil for 4-6 minutes per side, depending on the desired doneness. Let the steak rest for 5 minutes before slicing.

**Cook Barley:**

1. **Boil Broth or Water:** In a medium saucepan, bring vegetable broth or water to a boil. Add the pearl barley, cover, and reduce heat to low. Simmer for 30-40 minutes until the barley is tender and has absorbed most of the liquid.
2. **Season Barley:** Drain any excess liquid and transfer the barley to a bowl. Stir in olive oil, lemon zest, black pepper, and salt (if allowed). Add chopped parsley and mix well. **Assemble Plates and Serve.**

# Zucchini Lasagna with Ricotta

**Preparation Time:** 20 minutes • **Cooking Time:** 40 minutes • **Servings:** 4

### Ingredients:

- 3-4 medium zucchinis, sliced lengthwise into thin strips
- 2 tbsp (30 ml) olive oil
- 1 cup (240 g) ricotta cheese
- 1 cup (120 g) shredded mozzarella cheese
- ½ cup (60 g) grated Parmesan cheese
- 2 eggs, lightly beaten
- 2 tsp (10 ml) dried oregano
- 1 tsp (5 ml) black pepper
- Pinch of salt (if allowed)
- 2 cups (480 ml) tomato sauce (low-sodium if available)
- 2 garlic cloves, minced
- 2 tbsp (30 g) chopped fresh basil or parsley

**Nutritional Values (per serving):** Calories: 220 Protein: 14 g Carbohydrates: 8 g Fat: 14 g Sodium: 140 mg Potassium: 150 mg Phosphorus: 90 mg

### Procedure:

**Prepare Zucchini:**

1. **Preheat Oven:** Preheat the oven to 375°F (190°C).
2. **Slice Zucchini:** Slice the zucchinis lengthwise into thin strips using a mandoline or a sharp knife. Lay the strips on a paper towel to remove excess moisture.

**Prepare Cheese Mixture:**

1. **Mix Cheeses:** In a bowl, combine ricotta cheese, shredded mozzarella, grated Parmesan, eggs, oregano, black pepper, and salt (if allowed). Mix well until fully incorporated.

**Assemble Lasagna:**

1. **Spread Sauce:** Spread a layer of tomato sauce evenly on the bottom of a baking dish.
2. **Layer Ingredients:** Place a layer of zucchini strips over the sauce. Spoon some of the cheese mixture on top of the zucchini. Add another layer of tomato sauce over the cheese. Repeat the layers until all ingredients are used, finishing with a layer of sauce.
1. **Bake:** Cover the baking dish with foil and bake for 25-30 minutes until the zucchini is tender. Remove the foil and bake for another 5-10 minutes until the top is golden and bubbly. **Garnish & Serve.**

# Ratatouille with Couscous

- **Preparation Time:** 15 minutes
- **Cooking Time:** 35 minutes
- **Servings:** 4

**Ingredients:**

**Ratatouille:**

- 2 tbsp (30 ml) olive oil
- 1 medium onion, diced
- 2 garlic cloves, minced
- 1 medium eggplant, diced
- 2 medium zucchinis, diced
- 1 red bell pepper, diced
- 1 yellow bell pepper, diced
- 2 cups (480 ml) crushed tomatoes
- 1 tsp (5 ml) dried thyme
- 1 tsp (5 ml) dried oregano
- 1 tsp (5 ml) black pepper
- Pinch of salt (if allowed)
- 2 tbsp (30 g) chopped fresh basil

**Couscous:**

- 1 cup (180 g) couscous
- 1½ cups (360 ml) low-sodium vegetable broth or water
- 1 tbsp (15 ml) olive oil
- 1 tsp (5 ml) lemon juice
- ½ tsp (2.5 ml) black pepper
- Pinch of salt (if allowed)

**Nutritional Values (per serving):** Calories: 230 Protein: 6 g Carbohydrates: 32 g Fat: 8 g Sodium: 90 mg Potassium: 180 mg Phosphorus: 70 mg

**Procedure:**

**Cook Ratatouille:**

1. **Sauté Onion & Garlic:** In a large skillet, heat olive oil over medium heat. Add diced onion and garlic, and sauté for 5 minutes until softened.
2. **Cook Vegetables:** Add the diced eggplant, zucchinis, and bell peppers. Cook for 10 minutes, stirring occasionally, until the vegetables are softened.
3. **Add Tomatoes & Seasoning:** Stir in crushed tomatoes, thyme, oregano, black pepper, and salt (if using). Reduce heat to low and let it simmer for 20 minutes until the vegetables are tender.
4. **Finish with Basil:** Stir in the chopped basil just before serving.

**Prepare Couscous:**

**Boil Broth or Water:** In a medium saucepan, bring vegetable broth or water to a boil. Stir in the couscous, cover, and remove from heat. Let it sit for 5 minutes.

**Assemble Plates**

## Roasted Vegetable Frittata with Baby Spinach

- **Preparation Time:** 15 minutes
- **Cooking Time:** 30 minutes
- **Servings:** 4

### Ingredients:

- 2 tbsp (30 ml) olive oil
- 1 medium red bell pepper, diced
- 1 medium zucchini, diced
- 1 medium onion, diced
- 2 cups (60 g) baby spinach, roughly chopped
- 8 large eggs
- ¼ cup (60 ml) low-fat milk
- 1 tsp (5 ml) black pepper
- Pinch of salt (if allowed)
- ¼ cup (30 g) crumbled feta cheese (optional)
- 2 tbsp (30 g) chopped fresh parsley

**Nutritional Values (per serving):** Calories: 190 Protein: 10 g Carbohydrates: 8 g Fat: 14 g Sodium: 110 mg Potassium: 150 mg Phosphorus: 80 mg

### Procedure:

**Roast Vegetables:**

1. **Preheat Oven:** Preheat the oven to 400°F (200°C).
2. **Season & Roast Vegetables:**
   - Toss the diced bell pepper, zucchini, and onion with 1 tbsp olive oil, black pepper, and salt (if allowed).
   - Spread them evenly on a baking sheet and roast for 15 minutes until tender and lightly browned.

**Prepare Frittata Mixture:**

1. **Whisk Eggs:** In a large bowl, whisk the eggs and milk until well combined. Stir in the roasted vegetables, chopped spinach, and feta cheese (if using). Adjust seasoning to taste.

**Cook Frittata:**

1. **Preheat Skillet:** In a large oven-safe skillet, heat 1 tbsp olive oil over medium heat.
2. **Add Egg Mixture:** Pour the egg mixture into the skillet and cook undisturbed for 5-7 minutes until the edges begin to set.

3. **Bake Frittata:** Transfer the skillet to the preheated oven and bake for 10-12 minutes until the frittata is fully set.

**Garnish & Serve:** Let the frittata cool for a few minutes before slicing.

## Spaghetti Squash with Turkey Bolognese Sauce

**Preparation Time:** 20 minutes • **Cooking Time:** 40 minutes • **Servings:** 4

### Ingredients:

**Spaghetti Squash:**

- 1 medium spaghetti squash
- 2 tbsp (30 ml) olive oil
- ½ tsp (2.5 ml) black pepper
- Pinch of salt (if allowed)

**Turkey Bolognese Sauce:**

- 1 tbsp (15 ml) olive oil
- 1 lb (450 g) ground turkey
- 1 medium onion, diced
- 2 garlic cloves, minced
- 1 carrot, diced
- 1 celery stalk, diced
- 1 can (14 oz or 400 g) crushed tomatoes
- 2 tbsp (30 ml) tomato paste
- 1 tsp (5 ml) dried basil
- 1 tsp (5 ml) dried oregano
- 1 tsp (5 ml) black pepper
- Pinch of salt (if allowed)
- ¼ cup (30 g) grated Parmesan cheese (optional)
- 2 tbsp (30 g) chopped fresh parsley

**Nutritional Values (per serving):** Calories: 250 Protein: 22 g Carbohydrates: 20 g Fat: 9 g Sodium: 110 mg Potassium: 180 mg Phosphorus: 100 mg

### Procedure:

**Prepare Spaghetti Squash:**

1. **Preheat Oven:** Preheat the oven to 400°F (200°C).
2. **Season & Roast Squash:**
   - Cut the spaghetti squash in half lengthwise and remove the seeds.
   - Brush the inside of each half with olive oil and season with black pepper and salt (if allowed).
   - Place the squash halves cut-side down on a baking sheet and roast for 35-40 minutes until tender.

**Prepare Turkey Bolognese Sauce:**

1. **Sauté Vegetables:**
   - In a large skillet, heat olive oil over medium heat.
   - Add diced onion, garlic, carrot, and celery.
   - Sauté for 5-7 minutes until softened.

2. **Cook Turkey:**
   - Add the ground turkey to the skillet and cook for 5-7 minutes, breaking it apart with a spatula, until no longer pink.

3. **Simmer Sauce:**
   - Stir in crushed tomatoes, tomato paste, basil, oregano, black pepper, and salt (if allowed).
   - Reduce heat to low and simmer for 20 minutes until the sauce thickens.

**Serve:**

1. **Shred Spaghetti Squash:**
   - Once the spaghetti squash is roasted, use a fork to scrape out the flesh into long, spaghetti-like strands.
   - Divide the strands among four plates.

2. **Top with Sauce:**
   - Spoon the turkey Bolognese sauce over the spaghetti squash.
   - Garnish with grated Parmesan cheese (if using) and chopped parsley.
   - Serve warm.

# Snacks

## Apple Slices with Almond Butter

- **Preparation Time:** 5 minutes
- **Servings:** 2

**Ingredients:**

- 2 medium apples, cored and sliced
- 4 tbsp (60 ml) almond butter
- 1 tsp (5 ml) ground cinnamon (optional)

**Nutritional Values (per serving):** Calories: 170 Protein: 4 g Carbohydrates: 24 g Fat: 8 g Sodium: 5 mg Potassium: 140 mg Phosphorus: 60 mg

**Procedure:**

1. **Core & Slice Apples:**
   - Core the apples and cut them into thin slices.
2. **Spread Almond Butter:**
   - Spread a generous layer of almond butter on each apple slice.
3. **Garnish & Serve:**
   - Sprinkle ground cinnamon over the top if desired.
   - Serve immediately as a quick snack.

**Batch Cooking and Meal Prepping Tips:**

- **Pre-Slice Apples:** Slice apples ahead of time and toss with a bit of lemon juice to prevent browning.
- **Portion Control:** Divide almond butter into small containers for easy dipping on the go.
- **Customization:** Experiment with different toppings like shredded coconut or chopped nuts for added flavor.

## Sliced Bell Peppers with Hummus

- **Preparation Time:** 5 minutes
- **Servings:** 2

**Ingredients:**

- 1 red bell pepper, cored and sliced
- 1 yellow bell pepper, cored and sliced
- ½ cup (120 g) hummus

**Nutritional Values (per serving):**

- Calories: 140
- Protein: 5 g
- Carbohydrates: 17 g
- Fat: 6 g
- Sodium: 120 mg
- Potassium: 200 mg
- Phosphorus: 60 mg

**Procedure:**

1. **Slice Bell Peppers:**
    - Core the bell peppers and cut them into thin strips.
2. **Serve with Hummus:**
    - Place the sliced bell peppers on a plate with a serving of hummus.
    - Enjoy as a healthy and colorful snack.

**Batch Cooking and Meal Prepping Tips:**

- **Pre-Slice Peppers:** Slice the bell peppers ahead of time and store them in an airtight container in the fridge for up to 3 days.
- **Portion Hummus:** Divide the hummus into small containers for easy dipping on the go.

- **Flavor Variety:** Experiment with different hummus flavors, like roasted red pepper or garlic, for a varied taste.

## Cucumber Rounds with Yogurt-Based Dip

- **Preparation Time:** 10 minutes
- **Servings:** 2

Ingredients:

Cucumber Rounds:

- 1 large cucumber, sliced into rounds

Yogurt-Based Dip:

- ½ cup (120 g) plain Greek yogurt
- 1 tsp (5 ml) lemon juice
- 1 tsp (5 ml) dried dill
- ½ tsp (2.5 ml) garlic powder
- ¼ tsp (1.25 ml) black pepper
- Pinch of salt (if allowed)

**Nutritional Values (per serving):** Calories: 80 Protein: 5 g Carbohydrates: 8 g Fat: 3 g Sodium: 60 mg Potassium: 180 mg Phosphorus: 40 mg

Procedure:

Prepare Cucumber Rounds:

1. **Slice Cucumber:** Cut the cucumber into thin rounds and arrange them on a serving plate.

Make Dip:

1. **Mix Ingredients:** In a bowl, combine Greek yogurt, lemon juice, dried dill, garlic powder, black pepper, and salt (if using). Mix well to combine.

Serve:

1. **Arrange & Serve:**
   - Place the yogurt-based dip in a small bowl alongside the cucumber rounds.
   - Serve immediately as a refreshing snack.

**Batch Cooking and Meal Prepping Tips:**

- **Portion Dip:** Divide the yogurt-based dip into small containers for easy dipping on the go.

## Trail Mix with Unsalted Seeds and Dried Apples

- **Preparation Time:** 5 minutes
- **Servings:** 4

**Ingredients:**

- ½ cup (75 g) unsalted sunflower seeds
- ½ cup (75 g) unsalted pumpkin seeds
- ½ cup (75 g) dried apples, diced
- ¼ cup (40 g) dried cranberries or raisins
- ¼ cup (40 g) unsweetened coconut flakes

**Nutritional Values (per serving):**

- Calories: 160
- Protein: 4 g
- Carbohydrates: 20 g
- Fat: 8 g
- Sodium: 5 mg
- Potassium: 120 mg
- Phosphorus: 70 mg

**Procedure:**

1. **Mix Ingredients:**
    - In a large bowl, combine the unsalted sunflower seeds, pumpkin seeds, dried apples, dried cranberries or raisins, and coconut flakes.
    - Mix well to distribute all ingredients evenly.
2. **Portion & Serve:**
    - Divide the trail mix into individual servings or a large airtight container.
    - Serve as a snack or pack for on-the-go eating.

**Batch Cooking and Meal Prepping Tips:**

- **Store Properly:** Store the trail mix in an airtight container for up to 2 weeks to maintain freshness.
- **Customize Mix:** Adjust ingredient proportions or substitute other unsalted seeds, dried fruits, or nuts based on personal preferences.

## Celery Sticks with Cottage Cheese

- **Preparation Time:** 5 minutes
- **Servings:** 2

**Ingredients:**

- 4 large celery stalks, washed and cut into sticks
- ½ cup (120 g) low-fat cottage cheese
- ¼ tsp (1.25 ml) black pepper
- Pinch of salt (if allowed)

**Nutritional Values (per serving):**

- Calories: 60
- Protein: 5 g
- Carbohydrates: 8 g
- Fat: 1 g
- Sodium: 80 mg
- Potassium: 150 mg
- Phosphorus: 40 mg

**Procedure:**

1. **Prepare Celery:**
   - Wash the celery stalks thoroughly and cut them into sticks.
2. **Season Cottage Cheese:**
   - In a small bowl, mix the cottage cheese with black pepper and salt (if allowed).
3. **Serve:**
   - Arrange the celery sticks on a plate and serve them with the seasoned cottage cheese.
   - Use the celery sticks as dippers for a crunchy snack.

**Batch Cooking and Meal Prepping Tips:**

- **Pre-Cut Celery:** Wash and cut the celery sticks ahead of time, storing them in an airtight container in the fridge for up to 2 days.
- **Portion Cottage Cheese:** Divide cottage cheese into small containers for easy dipping during the week.

## Fresh Pineapple Chunks

- **Preparation Time:** 10 minutes
- **Servings:** 2

**Ingredients:**

- 1 medium fresh pineapple, peeled and cored

**Nutritional Values (per serving):**

- Calories: 80
- Protein: 1 g
- Carbohydrates: 21 g
- Fat: 0 g
- Sodium: 2 mg
- Potassium: 180 mg
- Phosphorus: 14 mg

**Procedure:**

1. **Peel & Core Pineapple:**
   - Cut off the top and bottom of the pineapple.
   - Stand it upright and carefully slice off the outer skin, cutting deep enough to remove the eyes.
   - Cut the pineapple lengthwise into four quarters, remove the core from each quarter, and then cut into bite-sized chunks.
2. **Serve:**
   - Place the pineapple chunks in a bowl or on a plate and serve fresh.

**Batch Cooking and Meal Prepping Tips:**

- **Portion Control:** Divide the pineapple chunks into individual servings for convenient snacking or use in smoothies.
- **Store Properly:** Store the pineapple chunks in an airtight container in the fridge for up to 3 days.

## Whole Wheat Crackers with Guacamole

- **Preparation Time:** 10 minutes
- **Servings:** 2

Ingredients:

Guacamole:

- 2 ripe avocados, peeled and pitted
- 2 tbsp (30 ml) lime juice
- ½ medium red onion, finely chopped
- 1 garlic clove, minced
- 1 small tomato, finely diced
- ¼ tsp (1.25 ml) black pepper
- Pinch of salt (if allowed)
- 2 tbsp (30 g) chopped fresh cilantro

Crackers:

- 12 whole wheat crackers

**Nutritional Values (per serving):** Calories: 180 Protein: 3 g Carbohydrates: 20 g Fat: 12 g Sodium: 80 mg Potassium: 250 mg Phosphorus: 50 mg

Procedure:

Prepare Guacamole:

1. **Mash Avocados:** In a medium bowl, mash the avocados with a fork until smooth.
2. **Mix Ingredients:**
   - Stir in lime juice, chopped red onion, minced garlic, diced tomato, black pepper, and salt (if allowed).
   - Add the chopped cilantro and mix well to combine.
   - Adjust seasoning to taste.

Serve:

1. **Arrange & Serve:**

- Arrange the whole wheat crackers on a plate with a bowl of guacamole.
- Serve as a quick snack or appetizer.

**Batch Cooking and Meal Prepping Tips:**

- **Store Guacamole:** Keep the guacamole in an airtight container with plastic wrap pressed directly on the surface to prevent browning.

## Carrot Sticks with Tahini

- **Preparation Time:** 5 minutes
- **Servings:** 2

**Ingredients:**

- 4 large carrots, peeled and cut into sticks
- ¼ cup (60 ml) tahini
- 1 tbsp (15 ml) lemon juice
- 1 tsp (5 ml) ground cumin
- ½ tsp (2.5 ml) black pepper
- Pinch of salt (if allowed)

**Nutritional Values (per serving):**

- Calories: 120
- Protein: 4 g
- Carbohydrates: 14 g
- Fat: 6 g
- Sodium: 40 mg
- Potassium: 180 mg
- Phosphorus: 40 mg

**Procedure:**

1. **Prepare Carrot Sticks:**
   - Peel the carrots and cut them into sticks.
2. **Make Tahini Dip:**
   - In a small bowl, mix the tahini, lemon juice, cumin, black pepper, and salt (if allowed) until well combined.
3. **Serve:**
   - Arrange the carrot sticks on a plate and serve with the tahini dip.

**Batch Cooking and Meal Prepping Tips:**

- **Pre-Cut Carrots:** Peel and cut the carrots ahead of time, storing them in an airtight container in the fridge for up to 3 days.
- **Portion Tahini Dip:** Divide the tahini dip into small containers for easy dipping during the week.

## Air-Popped Popcorn with Paprika

- **Preparation Time:** 5 minutes
- **Cooking Time:** 5 minutes
- **Servings:** 2

**Ingredients:**

- ½ cup (100 g) popcorn kernels
- 1 tsp (5 ml) olive oil (optional)
- 1 tsp (5 ml) smoked paprika
- ½ tsp (2.5 ml) black pepper
- Pinch of salt (if allowed)

**Nutritional Values (per serving):** Calories: 120 Protein: 3 g Carbohydrates: 24 g Fat: 2 g Sodium: 30 mg Potassium: 50 mg Phosphorus: 40 mg

**Procedure:**

1. **Pop Kernels:**
    - In an air popper, add the popcorn kernels and pop them according to the manufacturer's instructions.
2. **Season Popcorn:**
    - In a large mixing bowl, drizzle olive oil over the popped popcorn (if using).
    - Sprinkle smoked paprika, black pepper, and salt (if allowed) over the popcorn.
    - Toss gently to coat evenly.
3. **Serve:**
    - Divide the seasoned popcorn into individual bowls or store it in an airtight container for later snacking.

**Batch Cooking and Meal Prepping Tips:**

- **Store Properly:** Keep popcorn in an airtight container to maintain freshness.

- **Flavor Variety:** Experiment with different seasonings like cumin or chili powder for a flavor twist.

### Rice Cakes with Sunflower Seed Butter and Pear Slices

- **Preparation Time:** 5 minutes
- **Servings:** 2

Ingredients:

- 4 rice cakes
- 4 tbsp (60 ml) sunflower seed butter
- 1 ripe pear, cored and thinly sliced
- 1 tsp (5 ml) ground cinnamon (optional)

**Nutritional Values (per serving):** Calories: 180 Protein: 4 g Carbohydrates: 30 g Fat: 7 g Sodium: 20 mg Potassium: 110 mg Phosphorus: 50 mg

Procedure:

1. **Spread Sunflower Seed Butter:** Spread a generous layer of sunflower seed butter on each rice cake.
2. **Top with Pear Slices:** Arrange pear slices evenly over the sunflower seed butter on each rice cake.
3. **Garnish & Serve:**
    - Sprinkle ground cinnamon over the top if desired.
    - Serve immediately as a light snack.

Batch Cooking and Meal Prepping Tips:

- **Pre-Slice Pears:** Slice pears ahead of time and toss them in lemon juice to prevent browning.
- **Portion Sunflower Seed Butter:** Divide the sunflower seed butter into small containers for easy assembly and dipping.
- **Flavor Variety:** Experiment with other seed or nut butters for different flavors.

# Drink Recipes

## Blueberry Banana Smoothie with Almond Milk

- **Preparation Time:** 5 minutes
- **Servings:** 2

**Ingredients:**

- 1 cup (150 g) frozen blueberries
- 1 ripe banana, sliced
- 1½ cups (360 ml) unsweetened almond milk
- 1 tbsp (15 ml) ground flaxseed
- 1 tsp (5 ml) honey or maple syrup (optional)

**Nutritional Values (per serving):** Calories: 120 Protein: 3 g Carbohydrates: 25 g Fat: 3 g Sodium: 60 mg Potassium: 200 mg Phosphorus: 40 mg

**Procedure:**

1. **Combine Ingredients:** In a blender, add frozen blueberries, banana slices, almond milk, ground flaxseed, and honey or maple syrup (if using).
2. **Blend Smoothie:**
   - Blend on high until the mixture is smooth and creamy.
   - If the consistency is too thick, add more almond milk.
3. **Serve:** Pour the smoothie into two glasses and serve immediately.

**Batch Cooking and Meal Prepping Tips:**

- **Pre-Portion Fruit:** Slice bananas and portion frozen blueberries into bags or containers for quick smoothie preparation.
- **Customize Flavor:** Experiment with adding other fruits like strawberries or mango to create new flavors.

## Strawberry Basil Lemonade

- **Preparation Time:** 10 minutes
- **Servings:** 4

Ingredients:

- 1 cup (150 g) fresh strawberries, hulled and chopped
- 2 tbsp (30 g) honey or sugar (optional)
- ¾ cup (180 ml) lemon juice (from about 3-4 lemons)
- 4 cups (960 ml) cold water
- ¼ cup (15 g) fresh basil leaves, torn
- Ice cubes

**Nutritional Values (per serving):** Calories: 60 Protein: 0 g Carbohydrates: 15 g Fat: 0 g Sodium: 5 mg Potassium: 70 mg Phosphorus: 10 mg

Procedure:

1. **Prepare Strawberry Puree:**
   - In a blender, add the chopped strawberries and honey or sugar (if using).
   - Blend until smooth.
2. **Mix Lemonade:**
   - In a large pitcher, combine the strawberry puree, lemon juice, and cold water.
   - Stir well to mix.
3. **Add Basil:**
   - Add the torn basil leaves to the pitcher and stir gently.
4. **Serve:**

- Fill glasses with ice cubes and pour the lemonade over the ice.
- Garnish with extra basil leaves if desired and serve immediately.

**Batch Cooking and Meal Prepping Tips:**

- **Customize Sweetness:** Adjust the sweetness by adding or reducing honey or sugar based on preference.
- **Flavor Variety:** Experiment with adding mint leaves or cucumber slices for a twist on flavor.

## Pineapple Mint Iced Tea

- **Preparation Time:** 10 minutes
- **Steeping Time:** 10 minutes
- **Servings:** 4

Ingredients:

- 4 cups (960 ml) water
- 4 black tea bags
- 1 cup (240 ml) pineapple juice
- 1 tbsp (15 ml) honey or sugar (optional)
- ¼ cup (15 g) fresh mint leaves, torn
- Ice cubes

**Nutritional Values (per serving):** Calories: 40 Protein: 0 g Carbohydrates: 10 g Fat: 0 g Sodium: 5 mg Potassium: 20 mg Phosphorus: 10 mg

**Procedure:**

1. **Brew Tea:**
    - In a medium saucepan, bring water to a boil.
    - Remove from heat and add the tea bags.
    - Steep for 10 minutes, then discard the tea bags and let the tea cool.
2. **Mix Iced Tea:**
    - In a large pitcher, combine the cooled tea, pineapple juice, and honey or sugar (if using).
    - Stir until well mixed.
3. **Add Mint:** Add the torn mint leaves to the pitcher and stir gently.
4. **Serve:**

- Fill glasses with ice cubes and pour the iced tea over the ice.
- Garnish with extra mint leaves if desired, and serve immediately.

**Batch Cooking and Meal Prepping Tips:**

- **Flavor Variety:** Add slices of lemon, lime, or fresh pineapple to the pitcher for more flavor options.

## Cucumber Lime Refresher

- **Preparation Time:** 10 minutes
- **Servings:** 4

**Ingredients:**

- 1 large cucumber, peeled and thinly sliced
- ½ cup (120 ml) lime juice (from about 4-5 limes)
- 4 cups (960 ml) cold water
- 1 tbsp (15 ml) honey or sugar (optional)
- Ice cubes
- Fresh mint leaves (optional)

**Nutritional Values (per serving):** Calories: 20 Protein: 0 g Carbohydrates: 5 g Fat: 0 g Sodium: 2 mg Potassium: 40 mg Phosphorus: 5 mg

**Procedure:**

1. **Mix Drink:**
    - In a large pitcher, combine sliced cucumber, lime juice, and cold water.
    - Add honey or sugar (if using) and stir until well mixed.
2. **Add Ice & Mint:**
    - Add ice cubes to the pitcher to chill the drink.
    - If desired, add a few fresh mint leaves for extra flavor.
3. **Serve:**
    - Pour the cucumber lime refresher into glasses over ice and garnish with additional mint leaves if desired.
    - Serve immediately as a cooling beverage.

**Batch Cooking and Meal Prepping Tips:**

- **Pre-Chill Ingredients:** Chill cucumber and lime juice before preparing for extra refreshment.
- **Flavor Variety:** Experiment with adding lemon slices, basil leaves, or other herbs for new flavor combinations.

## Apple Cinnamon Infused Water

- **Preparation Time:** 5 minutes
- **Infusion Time:** 1 hour
- **Servings:** 4

**Ingredients:**

- 1 large apple, cored and thinly sliced
- 2 cinnamon sticks
- 4 cups (960 ml) cold water
- Ice cubes

**Nutritional Values (per serving):** Calories: 10 Protein: 0 g Carbohydrates: 2 g Fat: 0 g Sodium: 2 mg Potassium: 20 mg Phosphorus: 5 mg

**Procedure:**

1. **Combine Ingredients:**
   - In a large pitcher, add apple slices and cinnamon sticks to the cold water.
   - Stir gently to mix.
2. **Infuse:** Let the water sit in the fridge for at least an hour, or overnight, to allow the flavors to infuse.
3. **Serve:**
   - Fill glasses with ice cubes and pour the infused water over the ice.
   - Serve immediately for a refreshing and lightly flavored drink.

**Batch Cooking and Meal Prepping Tips:**

- **Pre-Chill Ingredients:** Keep apples chilled before slicing to speed up the infusion process.

- **Store Properly:** Store the infused water in the fridge for up to 24 hours for maximum flavor.
- **Flavor Variety:** Add other fruits like lemon or pear slices to enhance the flavor profile.

## Raspberry Coconut Water Cooler

- **Preparation Time:** 5 minutes
- **Infusion Time:** 1 hour
- **Servings:** 4

Ingredients:

- 1 cup (150 g) fresh raspberries
- 4 cups (960 ml) coconut water
- Ice cubes
- Fresh mint leaves (optional)

**Nutritional Values (per serving):** Calories: 35 Protein: 0 g Carbohydrates: 8 g Fat: 0 g Sodium: 20 mg Potassium: 100 mg Phosphorus: 5 mg

Procedure:

1. **Combine Ingredients:**
   - In a large pitcher, add fresh raspberries to the coconut water.
   - Stir gently to combine.
2. **Infuse:**
   - Let the cooler sit in the fridge for at least an hour to allow the flavors to infuse.
3. **Serve:**
   - Fill glasses with ice cubes and pour the infused water over the ice.
   - Garnish with fresh mint leaves if desired, and serve immediately.

**Batch Cooking and Meal Prepping Tips:**

- **Pre-Chill Ingredients:** Keep raspberries chilled before adding them to the cooler for quicker infusion.

- **Store Properly:** Store the cooler in the fridge for up to 24 hours.
- **Flavor Variety:** Add lemon or lime slices to the cooler for an extra citrusy twist.

*Watermelon Lime Slush*

- **Preparation Time:** 5 minutes
- **Servings:** 2

**Ingredients:**

- 4 cups (600 g) watermelon, cubed and frozen
- ¼ cup (60 ml) lime juice (from about 2-3 limes)
- 1 tbsp (15 ml) honey or sugar (optional)
- ½ cup (120 ml) cold water
- Fresh mint leaves (optional)

**Nutritional Values (per serving):** Calories: 45 Protein: 1 g Carbohydrates: 12 g Fat: 0 g Sodium: 2 mg Potassium: 150 mg Phosphorus: 5 mg

**Procedure:**

1. **Blend Ingredients:**
    - In a blender, add the frozen watermelon cubes, lime juice, honey or sugar (if using), and cold water.
    - Blend until the mixture becomes smooth and slushy.
2. **Serve:**
    - Pour the watermelon lime slush into glasses and garnish with fresh mint leaves if desired.
    - Serve immediately as a refreshing frozen beverage.

**Batch Cooking and Meal Prepping Tips:**

- **Pre-Freeze Watermelon:** Cube and freeze watermelon ahead of time for quicker slush preparation.
- **Flavor Variety:** Experiment by adding other fruits like strawberries or pineapple for extra flavors.

## Ginger Turmeric Tonic

- **Preparation Time:** 10 minutes
- **Cooking Time:** 10 minutes
- **Servings:** 4

**Ingredients:**

- 4 cups (960 ml) water
- 2-inch (5 cm) fresh ginger root, peeled and thinly sliced
- 1½ tsp (7.5 ml) ground turmeric or 1 tbsp (15 ml) fresh turmeric, grated
- 2 tbsp (30 ml) lemon juice
- 1 tbsp (15 ml) honey or maple syrup (optional)

**Nutritional Values (per serving):** Calories: 15 Protein: 0 g Carbohydrates: 4 g Fat: 0 g Sodium: 2 mg Potassium: 15 mg Phosphorus: 2 mg

**Procedure:**

1. **Boil Water:**
    - In a medium saucepan, bring water to a boil.
2. **Add Ingredients:**
    - Add the sliced ginger and turmeric to the boiling water.
    - Reduce heat and let it simmer for 10 minutes.
3. **Strain & Sweeten:**
    - Strain the tonic into a pitcher or bowl to remove the ginger and turmeric solids.
    - Stir in lemon juice and honey or maple syrup (if using).
4. **Serve:**
    - Serve the tonic warm, or chill it in the fridge for a refreshing cold drink.

**Batch Cooking and Meal Prepping Tips:**

- **Store Properly:** Keep the tonic in an airtight container in the fridge for up to 3 days.
- **Flavor Variety:** Add black pepper or cinnamon sticks for extra flavor.

### Mango Peach Smoothie with Coconut Water

- **Preparation Time:** 5 minutes
- **Servings:** 2

Ingredients:

- 1 cup (150 g) frozen mango chunks
- 1 cup (150 g) frozen peach slices
- 1½ cups (360 ml) coconut water
- 1 tsp (5 ml) honey or agave syrup (optional)

**Nutritional Values (per serving):** Calories: 70 Protein: 1 g Carbohydrates: 17 g Fat: 0 g Sodium: 25 mg Potassium: 100 mg Phosphorus: 10 mg

Procedure:

1. **Combine Ingredients:**
    - In a blender, combine frozen mango, frozen peach, coconut water, and honey or agave syrup (if using).
2. **Blend Smoothie:**
    - Blend on high until smooth and creamy.
    - Adjust the consistency with more coconut water if needed.
3. **Serve:**
    - Pour the smoothie into glasses and serve immediately.

Batch Cooking and Meal Prepping Tips:

- **Pre-Portion Fruit:** Divide mango chunks and peach slices into small bags or containers to quickly prepare smoothies on the go.
- **Customize Flavor:** Add other fruits like pineapple or berries for a unique twist on the flavor.

## Herbal Tea Blend with Peppermint and Chamomile

- **Preparation Time:** 5 minutes
- **Steeping Time:** 5-10 minutes
- **Servings:** 4

**Ingredients:**

- 4 cups (960 ml) water
- 2 tbsp (30 g) dried peppermint leaves
- 2 tbsp (30 g) dried chamomile flowers
- Honey or agave syrup (optional)

**Nutritional Values (per serving):** Calories: 0-10 (depending on sweetener) Protein: 0 g Carbohydrates: 0 g (without sweetener) Fat: 0 g Sodium: 0 mg Potassium: 0 mg Phosphorus: 0 mg

**Procedure:**

1. **Boil Water:**
   - Bring water to a boil in a medium saucepan or kettle.
2. **Steep Herbs:**
   - In a teapot or heatproof bowl, add dried peppermint leaves and dried chamomile flowers.
   - Pour boiling water over the herbs, cover, and let it steep for 5-10 minutes.
3. **Strain & Sweeten:**
   - Strain the herbal tea into a pitcher or individual cups to remove the leaves and flowers.
   - Sweeten with honey or agave syrup if desired.

4. **Serve:**
    - Serve warm, or chill the tea in the fridge for a refreshing cold drink.

**Batch Cooking and Meal Prepping Tips:**

- **Store Properly:** Keep the tea in the fridge for up to 2 days in an airtight container.
- **Customize Flavor:** Add dried lemon balm, lavender, or ginger root to the blend for a unique twist.

*Download your bonus via the QR code below!*

Your review is valuable: share your experience and help us improve by offering more and more useful content.

Thank you for your support!